S0-BYB-320

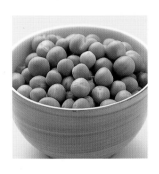

Power
Food

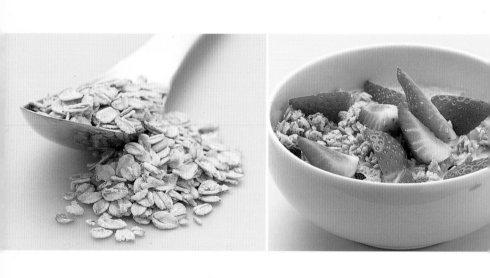

Power
Food

Janette Marshall

hamlyn

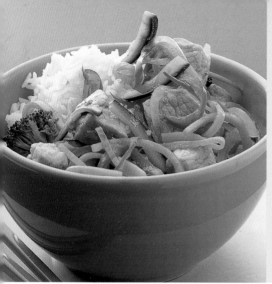

A Pyramid Paperback from Hamlyn

First published in Great Britain in 2004 by
Hamlyn, a division of Octopus Publishing Group Ltd
2–4 Heron Quays, London E14 4JP

Copyright text and recipes © Janette Marshall 2002
Copyright book design © Octopus Publishing Group Ltd 2002

All rights reserved. No part of this work may be reproduced or utilized in any form or by any means, electronic or mechanical, including photocopying, recording or by any information storage and retrieval system, without the prior written permission of the publisher.

ISBN 0 600 61087 X

A CIP catalogue record for this book is available from the British Library

Printed and bound in China

10 9 8 7 6 5 4 3 2 1

Contents

Power Food is meant to be used as a general reference and recipe book. While the author believes the information and recipes it contains are beneficial to health, the book is in no way intended to replace medical advice. You are therefore urged to consult your health-care professional about specific medical complaints and the use of alternative medicine.

While all reasonable care has been taken during the preparation of this edition, neither the publisher, editors, nor the author can accept responsibility for any consequences arising from the use of the information within.

notes

1. Standard level spoon measurements are used in all recipes.
   1 tablespoon = one 15 ml spoon
   1 teaspoon = one 5 ml spoon

2. Both metric and imperial measurements have been given in all recipes. Use one set of measurements only, and not a mixture of both.

3. Eggs should be large unless otherwise stated. The Department of Health advises that eggs should not be consumed raw. This book contains dishes made with raw or lightly cooked eggs. It is prudent for more vulnerable peoplie such as pregnant and nursing mothers, invalids, the elderly, babies and young children to avoid uncooked or lightly cooked dishes made with eggs. Once prepared, these dishes should be kept refrigerated and used promptly.

4. Ovens should be pre-heated to the specified temperature – if using a fan-assisted oven, follow the manufacturer's instructions for adjusting the time and the temperature.

5. This book includes dishes made with nuts and nut derivatives. It is advisable for customers with known allergic reactions to nuts and nut derivatives and those who may be potentially vulnerable to these allergies, such as pregnant and nursing mothers, invalids, the elderly, babies and children to avoid dishes made with nuts and nut oils. It is also prudent to check the labels of pre-prepared ingredients for the possible inclusion of nut derivatives.

what are power foods?

Power foods give you energy and strength. Eating them results in increased vitality, which enables you to live life more fully. Power foods fight fatigue and boost immunity, helping to keep you fit and healthy.

the power to enjoy your food

While there is a place in the diet for all of the foods that you enjoy, some are undeniably richer than others in beneficial and essential nutrients – vitamins, minerals and naturally occurring phytochemicals. By eating more of these foods and by ensuring you have the correct proportion of different foods in your diet, you will have greater energy, endurance and stamina, enjoying more power from the foods you eat. Numerous studies show that diets rich in certain foods can be equated with better health and the absence of particular diseases.

In this book, you will learn more about the properties of these foods and how to use them in delicious and exciting recipes. There is great emphasis on complex carbohydrates – also called starchy foods or wholegrain foods – and fruit and vegetables, because these are the most potent sources of energy. Consumption of whole grains, for example, helps maintain a healthy heart and healthy digestive and immune systems. Wholegrain foods boost fibre intake, which helps to promote regular bowel movements and keep your intestines disease-free. And a low-fat diet rich in whole grains and other plant foods improves blood sugar control, important to combat the rising incidence of diabetes.

You will also learn more about fruit and vegetables, which are a vital source of antioxidants, in the form of vitamins, minerals, phytochemicals and other naturally occurring substances in plants. Antioxidants are needed to improve immunity and to protect you from the diseases that can disempower you.

not by food alone

There are other aspects of lifestyle that are beyond the remit of this book but which have a great impact on your power levels. The following are vitally important:

- taking enough exercise
- not smoking
- limiting alcohol and drug use, if applicable
- dealing with stress effectively

Being positive and happy can boost immunity and improve general well-being. Meditation is a technique that can be used to achieve this stress-free state of mind. Your positive attitude, your support network of family and friends, and the satisfaction you gain from your work, family life and other activities will also determine your power potential in life.

best foods for energy

One of the most important qualities of power foods is that they give you energy, and some foods are better at providing energy than others. The best source of energy is carbohydrate foods. **Carbohydrates** are one of the four main food groups.

The others are:

- **protein foods** which build muscle for physical power
- **fruit and vegetables** which provide essential nutrients for immunity and vitality
- **dairy foods** for calcium and other minerals to build and maintain strong bones and teeth

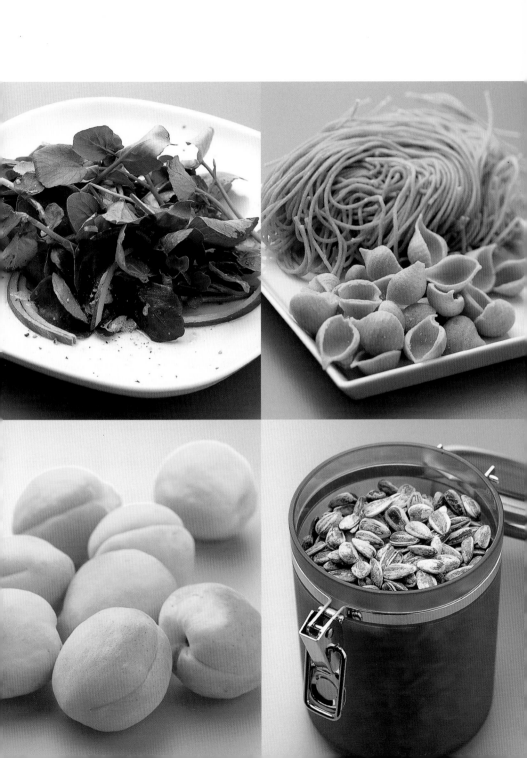

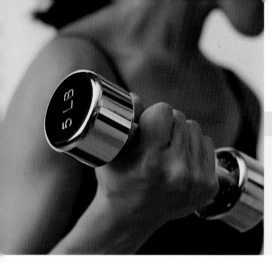

Power is the ability to do something – indeed, anything. It's a faculty of body or mind and it usually refers to the ability to do something with strength. It's about command and control. How does this translate to food and diet? It means that if you eat well, you are supplying your body with top-quality fuel so that it can function at full power, both physically and mentally.

the importance of the glycaemic index (GI)

The effect of different foods on blood-sugar levels is emerging as a powerful nutritional factor. This effect is measured by the glycaemic index (GI), which is a ranking of foods based on their effect on blood-sugar levels. Low GI means that a food breaks down slowly during digestion, releasing energy gradually into the bloodstream and resulting in a smaller rise in blood sugar. This is better for increasing your stamina and beneficial for health. High GI means that a food results in a larger rise in blood sugar.

Low GI is more desirable because it can:

• help control hunger, appetite and weight

• lower raised blood fats

• improve sensitivity to insulin

• help control diabetes

• possibly help prevent type 2 diabetes
  (the type that occurs later in life)

Studying the actual blood sugar response to hundreds of different foods on both healthy people and people with diabetes has helped scientists come up with a GI ranking of foods from 0 (good) to 100 (bad) that charts the effect of food on blood sugar levels. Low GI foods score 55 or below. Intermediate GI foods score between 55 and 70 and high GI foods more than 70.

Some of the results have been surprising particularly, for example, that some kinds of bread, potatoes and rice are digested quickly, whereas on the other hand certain mixed foods that contained sugar (ice-cream, some confectionery) did not produce as dramatic a rise in blood sugar as had been expected.

Pasta, white and wholemeal, made in the traditional way from durum wheat, has a low GI factor (30 to 50), with wholemeal pastas having the lower scores. This is because the durum wheat grain is very hard and the semolina, the starchy centre of the cracked grain, breaks into large particles which resist breakdown by enzymes during digestion. Pasta made from rice or vegetable flour or softer flour usually has a higher GI score. Of all the starchy staples, pasta (fresh or dried) has the lowest GI. The GI score of potatoes and rice varies between varieties, but not enough to be important in the overall diet.

Regardless of GI score, bread, potatoes, pasta and rice are all very valuable foods, and the wholemeal and brown versions are the most nutritious. Incidentally, the power foods peas, carrots and sweetcorn share the distinction of having the lowest GI among vegetables.

We have included the GI rating in the Power Content banner at the top of each Power Food entry. However, to date not all foods have been analysed for their GI rating.

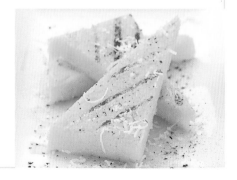

The world's staples are complex carbohydrate foods such as rice, pasta, bread, potatoes, starchy vegetables and cereals. At present, most people in the West do not eat enough starchy food for the balance of their diet to be right. There are practical ways to make more of starchy food.

Here are the main ones:

- Make bread, pasta, potatoes, or rice the main part of most meals.
- Serve larger portions of bread, pasta, rice and potatoes.
- Make more frequent use of noodles and bread made from other whole grains such as rice and buckwheat.
- Breakfast cereals can be enjoyed as a healthy snack at any time of the day, especially varieties that are fortified and whole grain – a great filler for hungry children after school.
- Use different varieties of rice, e.g. long-grain (brown or white) for pilaf, short-grain for paella, brown rice for salads, Arborio, Carnaroli or other speciality rices for risotto, wild rice with fish.
- Try sweet potato, plantain or yam instead of potato.

carbohydrate power foods

Many foods are a complicated mix of carbohydrates, protein, fats and various nutrients. However, there are also foods that are predominantly carbohydrate, or protein or fat.

The brain, heart and nervous system all need a constant supply of carbohydrates. Carbohydrates fuel your daily life; you use energy from carbohydrates to breathe, to think and to move.

There are two types of carbohydrate: starch and sugar. Starches and sugars are our main source of food energy. Fibre is built into the structure of complex carbohydrate (starchy) foods, so it is also described as a type of carbohydrate. These days fibre is called non-starch polysaccharides (NSP). There are many different types of NSP: two of the best-known examples are cellulose and pectin.

Complex carbohydrates or wholegrain foods are the most nutritious source of energy. They provide a steadier stream of energy than sugar because they break down slowly during digestion, releasing energy gradually into the bloodstream and resulting in a smaller rise of blood sugar. This is beneficial to health and maintains your power base for longer.

Sugars can occur naturally in fruit and vegetables,

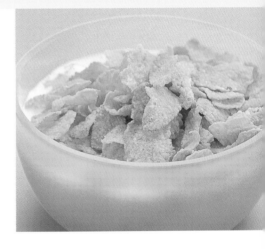

but when we talk about sugar we usually mean the refined stuff in the sugar bowl and in confectionery, biscuits, cakes and pastries. This type of sugar is regarded as 'empty calories' by nutritionists because it does not contribute any vitamins, minerals, NSP or other beneficial substances; it is purely calories and cannot match the benefits of complex carbohydrates. As starchy foods are broken down into simple sugars during digestion, in which form they enter the bloodstream to power all the body's cells, there is no nutritional need to eat sugar. However, neither is there

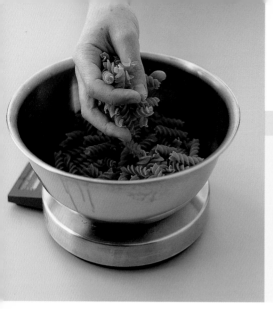

how much NSP (fibre) do you need?

The average person eats about 12 g (½ oz) of NSP a day. But 16 g (just over ½ oz) for women and 20 g (¾ oz) for men, would be better.

But don't go mad:
- 24 g (1 oz) a day is maximum for most people
- over 32 g (1½ oz) a day gives no further benefit

Eating wholemeal pasta is one way of increasing the NSP content of your diet.

any need to become obsessive about avoiding all sugar. Most people enjoy some sugary foods and, as part of a well-balanced diet, a small amount of sugary food is not a problem. The converse has been found to be true: people who obsessively avoid sugar (or other foods such as chocolate) can end up bingeing on it.

It seems paradoxical that slower release of energy results in greater power, but it does!

The slow, sustained release of energy from complex starchy foods is also due to their glycaemic index (GI).

other powers of starchy foods

While the GI index is a new concept, the knowledge that the NSP in starchy foods prevents constipation is not new. It does this by bulking (along with friendly bacteria, see page 16) and softening food waste as it passes through the gut. Helping the digestive system function better can prevent diverticular disease and help control some types of irritable bowel syndrome. Preventing constipation also helps to avoid haemorrhoids (piles) and varicose veins.

fibre confusion

Food labelling of fibre or NSP content is currently in a state of confusion. In the EU there are two methods of fibre analysis in use. The Englyst method measures only NSP and is a method also used by the Department of Health when recommending consumption of 18 g (½ oz) per day (see box above) – this enables consumers to keep track of healthy eating targets. There is also a method known as AOAC, which includes substances in addition to NSP (other types of saccharides, 'retrograded' starch, lignins and other substances). Food manufacturers are keen to use the AOAC method because it makes their foods look higher in fibre – and therefore healthier – than they are. So far, international agreement has not been reached on how to deal with this exploitation which can be seen, for example, on packs of certain breakfast cereals such as corn flakes.

why whole grains matter

The food as a whole is more important than isolated parts and nutrients (which is why vitamin supplements can never take the place of real food). Nutrients and other substances that are found in plant foods work together in powerful ways. Health benefits come from the way that all the elements interact with each other in the complete food.

Phytochemicals from plant foods are also powerful antioxidants, and when the diet is rich in them there is an association with improved health. When a grain is more refined, the level of these antioxidant substances is lower. Key antioxidants in whole grains (in addition to certain phytochemicals) include vitamin E and the trace element selenium.

Whole foods such as fruits, vegetables and whole grains deliver packages of nutrients and phytochemicals that may work synergistically (together) to protect health. NSP alone may lack the health-promoting properties found in whole grains.

Although it is not known how whole grains maintain health, several studies clearly show that regular consumption of them is beneficial. One recent study found that in a large group of women aged 55–69, eating at least one serving a day of wholegrain foods (mainly dark breads such as pumpernickel and wholegrain breakfast cereals) significantly improved their health compared with that of women who ate almost no wholegrain products.

starchy foods for a healthy heart and cancer protection

There are several theories as to how whole grains may help maintain a healthy heart. Whole grains are rich in vitamin E, which is now believed to be a cancer inhibitor by preventing the formation of carcinogens.

• Whole grains are also a source of other substances such as sterols and stanols, which have been shown to lower cholesterol.

• NSP is fermented by gut bacteria to make short-chain fatty acids that may help lower blood cholesterol. The soluble fibre found in grains such as oats also helps lower blood cholesterol by increasing cholesterol excretion from the body. This also protects against gallstones.

• Whole grains are a rich source of selenium, though the selenium content will depend on the soil where the grain was grown. Higher than average intakes of selenium (in supplement form) have generally been associated with a lower risk of cancer. This may be due to selenium working with an enzyme that protects

against oxidative tissue damage. At high levels, selenium can suppress potentially harmful cell proliferation, but be warned that too much can be toxic.

• A type of phytoestrogen (hormonally active plant compound) called lignans, found in whole grains, may protect against hormonal-related breast and prostate cancer. Refining eliminates the outer layers of the grain, where lignans are the most concentrated whereas whole grains include the lignan-rich outer layers.

anti-nutrients in whole grains

Whole grains also contain several substances that work against nutrients. These include phytates and other substances. Until recently, these substances were thought to have only negative nutritional consequences; however, some of them may act as cancer inhibitors. Phytic acid or phytates, for example, in bran can inhibit absorption of minerals such as iron that fight fatigue, which is why raw bran should not be added to food. However, as part of the whole grain, phytic acid is probably beneficial. Phytates do not make wholegrain

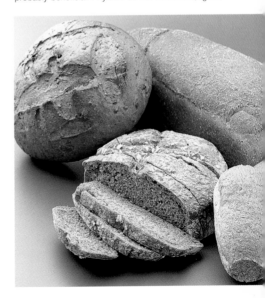

More familiar nutrients within starchy foods also help to boost vitality by releasing energy to the body.

Vitamin B1 (thiamin) Brown rice; peas, beans and other vegetables; fortified breakfast cereals; wholemeal breads and cereals; pork, bacon and liver.

Thiamin is essential for enzymes that convert food into fuel for the body. Also needed to transmit messages between brain and spinal cord.

Vitamin B2 (riboflavin) Liver, kidneys, meat; fortified breakfast cereals; some green vegetables; eggs; milk, cheese; yeast extracts.

Riboflavin also works with iron, vitamin B6 and folic acid. It is vital for releasing energy and is important for skin and eye health.

Vitamin B3 (niacin) Meat, poultry, oily fish; bread; potatoes; breakfast cereals; and can be synthesized from tryptophan (an essential amino acid).

Vital for energy from food to get into tissues and cells. Helps to maintain a healthy nervous and digestive system and essential for normal growth and for healthy skin.

Vitamin B6 (pyridoxine) Wholemeal bread; meat (especially liver and pork); fish; bananas; wheat bran; and fortified breakfast cereals.

Needed for the formation of haemoglobin in red blood cells, and therefore (like iron) prevents fatigue, tiredness and anaemia. Important too in protein metabolism; promotes healthy skin and is essential for the nervous system. Builds antibodies that help fight infection.

Iron Offal, red meat especially beef and pork; canned pilchards/sardines, fish, shellfish; wholegrain cereals; eggs, chicken; spinach, leafy green vegetables; fortified breakfast cereals.

Iron deficiency results in anaemia, but before iron intake becomes that low, symptoms of tiredness, lack of concentration and poor mental performance can also all be attributed to lack of iron. Iron is essential for the daily formation of haemoglobin in red blood cells that transport oxygen around the body.

Zinc Red meat, liver; shellfish (particularly oysters); pulses; wholemeal bread and other wholegrain cereals; pumpkin seeds.

Similar role to iron in preventing tiredness. Also an important component of many enzymes including superoxide dismutase (a powerful antioxidant enzyme that neutralizes potentially damaging free radicals). Required to aid growth; needed for immune cell function and for healthy hair, skin and nails.

Magnesium Green plants. Main dietary sources are unrefined cereals and vegetables, peanuts and wholemeal bread.

Needed for the formation in the body of many enzymes that release energy from food. Vital for the nervous system and muscle movement and for the formation of healthy bones and teeth.

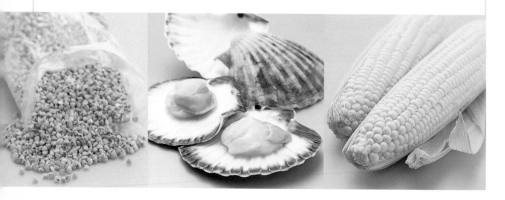

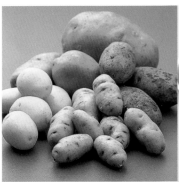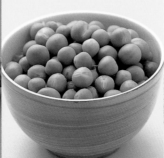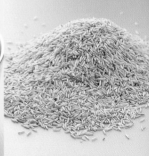

power foods as a source of folates

Good sources of folic acid (listed in order of content per serving):

- **15–50 mcg per average serving:** cooked soya beans, cauliflower, cooked chickpeas, potatoes, iceberg lettuce, oranges, peas, orange juice, parsnips, baked beans, wholemeal bread, cabbage, yogurt, white bread, eggs, brown rice, wholegrain pasta.

- **50–100 mcg per average serving:** cooked black-eye beans, Brussels sprouts, beef and yeast extracts, cooked kidney, kale, spinach, spring greens, broccoli and green beans.

food harmful because the body adjusts to absorb minerals when it has got used to a diet with a higher phytate content – for example, when changing from white bread and pasta to wholemeal.

starchy foods as providers of folic acid

Several breads and breakfast cereals are fortified with folic acid, and fortification of all flour with folic acid may soon be made law in the UK as it is in the US. Why is it so important? Folic acid is the vitamin supplement equivalent of folates, a member of the B vitamin complex found mainly in green leafy vegetables and wholegrain foods. It has been used as a supplement for pre-conceptual and pregnant women to protect their unborn babies against spina bifida and other neural tube defects. Now it is known that it also has protective powers against heart disease, which still claims or disables far too many lives prematurely.

the homocysteine story

We are familiar with the fact that a raised level of blood cholesterol increases a person's risk of heart disease, but it is now thought that a raised level of homocysteine may be more closely associated than cholesterol with increased risk of heart disease, stroke and vascular disease.

Homocysteine is an amino acid. It is converted in the body by the B vitamin folic acid to methionine, one of the body's essential building blocks of protein, and to other substances essential for brain function and making DNA. So, like cholesterol, homocysteine is essential for normal body function and structure. Problems with raised levels seem to occur when the diet does not provide enough folic acid and, less importantly, enough of two other B vitamins, B6 and B12, to clear the system of homocysteine.

Unlike raised blood cholesterol levels, which are quite hard to reduce (requiring weight loss, diet and exercise), homocysteine levels can be lowered quickly and easily by taking an extra 200 micrograms (mcg) of folic acid a day. This is 200 mcg more than the Reference Nutrient Intake (RNI – the amount thought to protect even those with higher than average needs). The RNI is 200 mcg per day for everyone aged 11 years and over, apart from pregnant and pre-conceptual women, who need 400 mcg or 0.4 mg per day. In addition to supplements, foods rich in folates can also be enjoyed regularly. There is no danger of overdosing.

To increase your intake without any difficulty, look out for starchy foods such as bread and bakery goods that are fortified with folic acid. Often the packaging is marked with a large blue 'f' symbol. Foods labelled 'contains extra folic acid' contain 100 mcg of folic acid per portion and those labelled 'contains folic acid' contain 33 mcg per portion.

Also remember, though, that homocysteine levels are only a part of the story. Heart disease and stroke have many other associated risk factors: smoking, high blood pressure, obesity, high salt and (saturated) fat intake, to name a few.

why eating less sugar might be better for you

It was mentioned earlier that starchy food is a more nutritious carbohydrate than sugary food because sugar lacks nutrients and NSP. There is another disadvantage of sugar, too. Habitually grazing on sugary foods may lead to a vicious circle of mood swings and sugar cravings. Sugar might give an instant energy boost, but it requires a lot of insulin and other hormones to clear the bloodstream of an influx of sugar, resulting in even lower blood-sugar levels after a sugary snack. These peaks and troughs can leave you feeling weak and wobbly. Starchy carbohydrate foods such as wholemeal bread or breakfast cereal; digestive biscuits or a cereal bar that is not too sugary; fruit such as bananas and dates – all are far better choices because they provide a steady stream of energy and they contain more vitamins and minerals. Of course you can enjoy chocolate, but eat it as a treat rather than a regular food.

Sugar is also more likely to cause dental decay (see page 41) than naturally occurring sugars found in fruit, wholegrain starchy foods and milk.

carbohydrate loading for sport

Athletes are great starchy food fans. Most élite athletes eat a high carbohydrate diet for a few days before an endurance event. This is called carbohydrate-loading. They also eat a starchy pre-event meal to boost their energy and endurance. The body turns the starches into glucose for the brain and to store in muscles and as glycogen in the liver. Starches are a better source of energy than sugar because they contain fibre, vitamins and minerals missing from sugars. Remember this after exercise, when a starchy snack, as opposed to sugary confectionery or drinks or fatty food, is better at replenishing depleted energy. A banana and some water is a lot less expensive than fashionable sports drinks – and does the job of rehydrating and boosting energy just as efficiently.

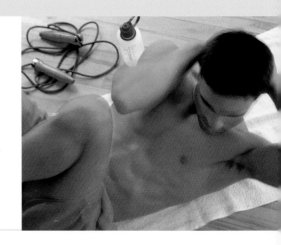

best foods to restore power and fight fatigue

Do you feel any of the following?

- tired all the time
- less fit than you used to be
- breathless when you exert yourself

These symptoms may be a sign of anaemia (see box, right), or the start of anaemia. If you suspect this, see your doctor. One-third of women have low iron stores, and it is particularly common for iron levels to be low after having a baby.

where to find iron-rich foods

Iron is most easily absorbed by the body from red meat, making it slightly more difficult for vegetarians. They can obtain iron from foods such as dark green vegetables, dried fruits, nuts, whole grains, pulses, seeds and fortified breakfast cereal. However, iron from plant foods is less readily available. Improve absorption by eating foods rich in vitamin C at the same time: oranges for pudding or a glass of orange juice with a meal, say.

what is anaemia?

Too little haemoglobin (the red pigment) in the blood causes anaemia. Haemoglobin transports oxygen to all parts of the body. If you are short of iron, your red blood cells contain less haemoglobin, so your body has to work harder to supply you with oxygen. This leaves you feeling tired, weak and short of breath. Teenagers, menstruating and pregnant women all have a high iron requirement, respectively for growth, to replace periodic losses and to make the larger volume of blood during pregnancy.

top scoring* antioxidant fruit and vegetables

Fruit Score:		Vegetable Score:	
Prunes	5,770	Kale	1,770
Raisins	2,830	Spinach	1,260
Blueberries	2,400	Brussels sprouts	980
Blackberries	2,036	Alfalfa sprouts	930
Strawberries	1,540	Broccoli	890
Raspberries	1,220	Beets	840
Plums	949	Red bell peppers	710
Oranges	750	Onions	450
Red grapes	739	Corn	400
Cherries	670	Aubergines	390
Kiwi fruit	602		
Pink grapefruit	483		

* The ORAC (short for Oxygen Radical Absorbance Capacity) score is a test-tube analysis that measures the total antioxidant power of food. The amounts given are ORAC units per 100 g/3½ oz food.

Source: Human Nutrition Research Center on Aging, Tufts University, Boston, US.

good sources of B vitamins

Meat also contains vitamin B12, needed to work with iron to prevent anaemia. Choose the leanest meat you can afford. Vegetarians can obtain vitamin B12 from fortified vegetarian products – some soy milk and 'yogurts', and meat substitutes such as textured vegetable protein. Other sources are yeast extract and fortified breakfast cereal.

Other B vitamins are also needed to work with iron to prevent anaemia. These include folic acid. Particularly good sources of folic acid are black-eye beans, the cabbage family, yeast extracts, pulses, vegetables and orange juice and eggs. Many breakfast cereals and some breads are fortified with folic acid – look out for the large blue 'f' symbol on packaging.

foods rich in vitamin C

Vitamin C is also needed to make healthy red blood cells and prevent tiredness and anaemia. Citrus fruits (including oranges, lemons, grapefruit), blackcurrants, other fruit and green vegetables are good sources.

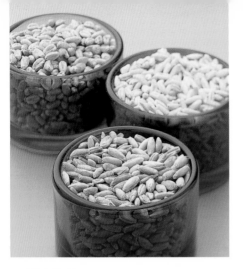

Eating the recommended 5 (or more) portions of fruit and vegetables a day will increase your intake of vitamin C and boost your immunity.

boost your power of immunity

Viral infections such as coughs, colds and particularly influenza can leave you run down and lacking energy. As prevention is always better than cure, try to boost your immunity. Eating lots of starchy carbohydrate foods and fruit and vegetables can help in ways other than the obvious contribution of vitamin C and B vitamins needed for a healthy immune system.

The less well-known contribution is through the NSP (fibre) content of complex carbohydrates. Foods such as bread, rice, pasta, potatoes, beans and pulses, vegetables, fruit, cereal and other grains contain non-digestible carbohydrates that reach the large intestine intact. There, friendly bacteria living in the mucus lining of the gut break down oligosaccharides and fructosaccharides, insulin and galactose. By fermenting these, bacteria produce a 'biomass' that bulks up body waste (more than half of stool weight is bacteria) to prevent constipation. Fermentation also produces substances such as butyrate. In the laboratory, butyrate

what kills friendly gut bacteria?

- antibiotics
- gastroenteritis
- laxatives
- radiotherapy
- chemotherapy
- severe deficiency of B vitamins
- emotional stress
- excessive physical activity, such as marathon-running
- ageing: the number of beneficial bacteria falls off dramatically after the age of 50

what can a healthy microflora do for you?

Lactobacillus casei and *bifido bacteria*:
- Limit travellers' diarrhoea and antibiotic-associated diarrhoea.
- Help reduce blood cholesterol levels by metabolizing fibre so it can remove cholesterol from the body.
- Protect against or suppress colon cancer.

Lactic acid, *Lactobacillus bulgaricus* and *Streptococcus thermophilus*:
- Assist the digestion of lactose (milk sugar), alleviating symptoms of lactose malabsorption in some people. Even if the bacteria do not

survive for long in the gut, the lactic acid they produce does.
- Metabolize the phytoestrogens from soy foods into their biologically active forms, giving protection against breast cancer.
- Synthesize B vitamins and folic acid, and vitamin K needed for blood clotting to prevent haemorrhage.
- Stimulate the immune system to increase antibody production. Antibodies protect against invasion by harmful bacteria and viruses.

quick snacks to boost your power levels

Enjoying a variety of food is the key to a well-balanced diet that will increase your power and vitality. Choosing from a diverse range of foods will ensure that you benefit from a wide range of nutrients and it also provides you with an exciting, colourful and tasty diet.

- wholemeal bread/toast, low-fat cheese
- jacket potato with cheese, baked beans
- toast, topped with cheese or beans or peanut butter
- wholemeal fruit bun/muffin, tea cake, malt loaf
- panforte (see page 102 or from Italian delicatessens)
- fruit salad
- fruit compote
- bananas, or any other fruit
- dried fruit (dates, apricots, peaches, pears)
- wholemeal sandwiches
- potato scones
- porridge
- breakfast cereal and skimmed milk or soya milk
- fruit yogurt and fromage frais
- unsalted nuts, or fruit and nut mixtures
- fruit cake

- samosas
- falafel
- tubs of salad (pasta, rice)
- eggs – boiled, poached, scrambled on toast
- hummus with pitta bread or vegetable sticks
- soup and roll
- fruit juice or 'smoothies' made from fruit juice and fruit purée
- yogurt drinks

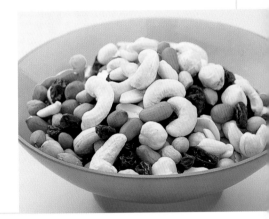

has been shown to cause cancer cells to commit suicide. Another effect of fermentation by beneficial bacteria is reduced risk of gallstones, and lower cholesterol levels.

Feeding experiments in healthy people have shown that by swapping as little as 15 g (3 teaspoons) of sugar in the diet for 15 g a day of oligosaccharides (obtained from the non-digestible parts of vegetables and fruit such as onions, garlic, artichoke, asparagus and banana), there is a dramatic change in the gut flora. With higher sugar intake, there are more bacteroides (potentially harmful gut bacteria), but with this small change in diet, beneficial bifido bacteria become dominant in 7 or 8 days.

snacking for extra power

Although often blamed for weight problems, on closer examination snacking, or more frequent eating, is not necessarily associated with obesity. Frequent eating among men does not correlate with body fatness and many snackers have a lower BMI (body mass index, a more reliable measure of weight problems than weight alone) than their counterparts. Studies show women and children who snack a lot to be no fatter than those who do not. Nibbling may help you stick to dietary guidelines and be beneficial to appetite control and health, whereas gorging does seem to contribute to obesity.

Eating low-fat snacks (sweet and/or savoury) can reduce total daily fat to help meet healthy eating targets.

power foods
in a healthy diet

There are four main food groups. Eaten in the right proportion, foods from these groups provide essential vitamins, minerals and other components for optimum health and vitality.

starchy carbohydrate foods eat 6–14 portions a day

An athlete might need 14 portions of starchy foods a day, whereas a sedentary woman would need only 5–6 portions per day.

portion guide:

- 45 g (2 oz) or 3 tablespoons breakfast cereal
- 30 g (1 oz) or 2 tablespoons muesli
- 1 slice of bread or toast

- 1 bread roll, bap or bun
- 1 small pitta bread, naan bread or chapatti
- 3 crackers or crispbreads
- 1 medium potato
- 30 g (2 oz) or 2 heaped tablespoons boiled rice
- 45 g (2 oz) or 3 heaped tablespoons boiled pasta
- 1 medium plantain or small sweet potato

vegetables and fruit eat 5–7 portions a day

At least 5 portions of vegetables and fruit per day are recommended – and there is more benefit in eating more. Choose a wide variety of all colours: orange, yellow, red, green.

portion guide:

- ½ avocado
- 4 fresh apricots
- 1 small banana
- 60 g (2½ oz) berry fruits (bilberries, blackcurrants, blueberries, gooseberries, raspberries, strawberries)
- 6 fresh or 4 dried dates
- 150 g (5 oz) stewed or canned fruit
- 1 small glass of fruit juice, 100 ml (3½ fl oz)
- 2 tablespoons of carrots
- 3 tablespoons of peas
- 1 corn on the cob
- 1 large or 6 cherry tomatoes
- 1 bunch of watercress

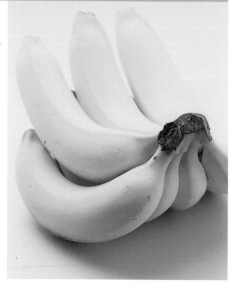

meat, fish and vegetarian protein alternatives eat 2–4 portions a day

Moderate amounts of fish, poultry, lean meat and vegetarian alternatives are needed for protein for growth and repair. Meat also provides magnesium, which promotes growth, healthy bones and skin, and iron, zinc and vitamin B12, which prevent anaemia. Choose lean meat – avoid pâté and meat pastes, pies, burgers, koftas, keemas, black and white pudding, faggots, frankfurters, haggis, luncheon meat, polony, salami, sausages and saveloys.

portion guide:

Government nutrition experts advise people to eat a maximum of 12–14 portions a week – and preferably less, to reduce the risk of colon cancer and possibly of breast, prostate and pancreatic cancer. Eating a lot of vegetables (and fruit) may ameliorate any risk among higher meat consumers. Meat-eaters are also advised to replace a couple of meat meals a week with fish; at least one of these should be oily fish such as herring or mackerel. Vegetarians will need 2–4 portions of vegetarian protein foods a day.

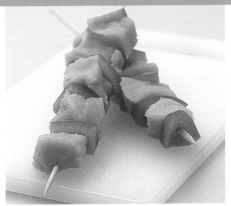

- 3 medium slices of beef, pork, ham, lamb, liver, kidney, chicken or oily fish, 45–75 g (2–3 oz)
- 125–150 g (4–5 oz) white fish (not fried in batter)
- 3 fish fingers
- 2 eggs (up to 4 a week)
- 200 g (7 oz) baked beans or other cooked pulses such as lentils
- 60 g (2½ oz) nuts, peanut butter or other nut products

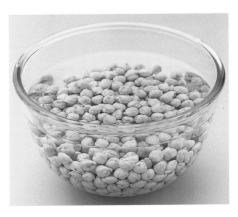

dairy foods eat 2–3 portions of lower-fat versions a day

Swapping to low-fat milk, yogurt, cheese, fromage frais and desserts will reduce fat in your diet, especially saturated fat. Dairy products are all good sources of calcium for strong bones and teeth. Bones and teeth are living matter, so people of all ages (not just children) have constant calcium needs. Dairy foods also provide protein for growth and repair, and vitamins A and D for eyes and teeth. While everyone over the age of 5 would benefit from lower-fat versions, infants and children up to the age of 2 need full-fat versions.

portion guide:
- 1 medium glass of milk, 200 ml (7 fl oz)
- 1 matchbox-sized piece of Cheddar-type cheese, 40 g (1½ oz)
- 1 small pot of yogurt, cottage cheese or fromage frais, 125 g (4 oz)

foods to eat in moderation only

A healthy, balanced diet does not mean avoiding certain foods altogether. Consume in moderation and enjoy an occasional treat.

foods containing fat eat 1–5 portions a day

Too much fat, and saturated fat in particular, increases the risk of heart disease by raising the level of harmful blood cholesterol. Diets high in fat also increase the risk of some cancers.

The maximum amount of fat needed depends on age, size and how active you are. But for most sedentary adults, to maintain a healthy weight women should eat no more than 70 g (just under 3 oz) of fat a day and men 90 g (just under 3½ oz).

portion guide to fats:

A portion of spreading fats and cooking oils is:

- 5 g (¼ oz) or 1 teaspoon margarine or butter
- 10 g (½ oz) or 2 teaspoons low-fat spread
- 5 ml (¼ fl oz) or 1 teaspoon cooking oil, fat or ghee

portion guide to fatty foods:

- 15 g (½ oz) or 1 tablespoon mayonnaise or vinaigrette (salad dressing)
- 15 ml (½ fl oz) or 1 tablespoon cream
- 1 packet of crisps

Other fatty foods include pastry, meat products, sausages, pâtés and fried foods.

Not all fats have the same effect:

Saturated fats (from meat and dairy produce and hydrogenated vegetable fats in margarine and processed foods) and trans fats, produced when vegetable oils are hydrogenated (hardened) to make margarine, raise levels of cholesterol and block production of essential long-chain fatty acids from vegetable and fish oils in the diet.

Polyunsaturates (from fish and from vegetable oils, except palm and coconut) are called essential fatty acids and must be provided by diet. There are two families: omega-6, from linoleic acid in vegetable oils (sunflower),

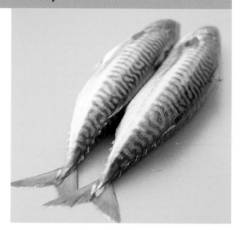

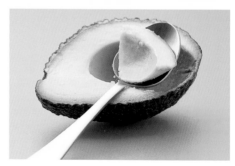

and omega-3, from linolenic acid in vegetable oils (soy and rape seed), in walnuts and in oily fish. The risk of heart attack is reduced by these fatty acids, which decrease the tendency of the blood to clot. (Their anti-inflammatory action also helps arthritis.)

Monounsaturates (from olive oil, groundnut and rapeseed oils, avocados, most nuts and some spreads) share the benefits of polyunsaturates.

Most people think of sugar as white or brown sugar, but sugar also includes honey, treacle, syrup, molasses, dextrose, glucose, fructose, maltose, corn syrups, glucose syrups and other industrial sugars added to processed foods.

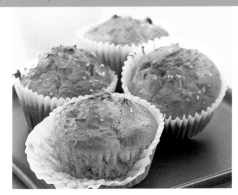

portion guide to sugar and sugary foods:

- 15 g (½ oz) or 1 tablespoon sugar
- 1 rounded teaspoon jam/honey
- 2 biscuits
- half a slice of cake or a doughnut or Danish pastry
- 1 small bar of chocolate
- 1 small tube or bag of sweets

salt

Salt is sodium chloride. Sodium is a mineral needed for a variety of body functions. All the sodium that most people need is naturally present in a well-balanced diet. The effect of eating too much salt, in combination with low potassium intake and being overweight, is rising blood pressure with age. High blood pressure increases the risk of strokes and heart disease.

How much salt and sodium? Currently we eat about 2–2½ teaspoons of salt per day. More than 80 per cent of this is from processed foods. We would probably benefit from eating less, 1 teaspoon (5 g).

beverages

alcohol

One unit of alcohol equals:

- ½ a pint of normal strength beer or lager
- 1 small glass of wine
- 1 pub measure of spirits
- 1 pub measure of fortified wine, e.g. sherry, Martini

Alcohol in a balanced diet

Moderate drinking, which means 2–3 units per day for women and 3–4 units per day for men (but not every day), is associated with reduced risk of heart disease and stroke among men and among women aged 45 and over. This equates to no more than 21 units a week for women and 28 for men. This is not the same as saying that drinking alcohol is good for you because it has many negative effects as well. Many experts are not happy with the 21 and 28 weekly units, which was revised upwards from 14 and 21 respectively.

other drinks

You should drink at least 6–8 cups, mugs or glasses of liquid (or around 1.5–2 litres) each day. Not all of that should be tea and coffee, because they contain stimulants (including caffeine) and are diuretic (making you lose water and nutrients in urine). Cola and other sweetened fizzy drinks also contain caffeine and sugar or artificial sweeteners and other non-nutritional additives. Water is the best drink for quenching thirst and hydrating the body. Other drinks include fruit juice, diluted juice, juice drinks, squash or cordials (but note that some of these contain only around 5 per cent juice, the rest being mainly water and sugar or additives – do not be fooled into thinking they are all fruit juice). There is a wide range of herb and fruit 'teas' available – these are not in fact tea, but just use the name generically as they are an infusion in hot water.

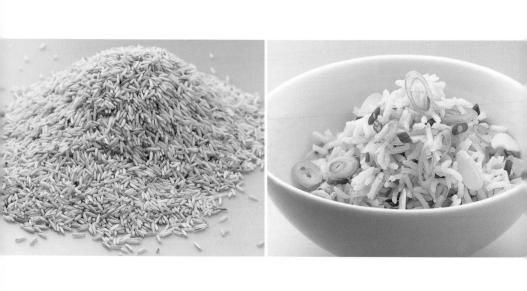

power foods & recipes

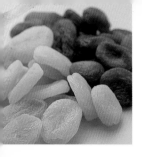

apricots

This fruit has been cultivated by the Chinese since 2000 BC and has subsequently been adopted throughout the world. Dried apricots from the Hunza region of Pakistan are reputed to contribute to the longevity of the inhabitants of that region.

POWER CONTENT

Vitamin C
NSP (fibre)
Iron
Potassium
Sorbitol
Beta-carotene
GI 57 (fresh)
GI 31 (dried)

PLUS POINTS

+ **High-fibre food (especially dried) for slow-release energy (like many other dried fruits, they make a good sports snack).**

+ **Fresh or dried, they contain beta carotene to neutralize the effect of damaging free radicals.**

+ **Dried apricots are a good source of iron to prevent tiredness and anaemia.**

The name apricot derives from the Roman word *praecox*, meaning early-ripening, because it fruits and ripens early in the summer. The apricot's velvety, blushing, downy skin and delicate aroma and colour have earned it a reputation as a sensuous fruit. Literature contains many romantic allusions to the apricot.

fresh and appealing

For the more pragmatic, apricots also have many appealing characteristics. The fresh fruit is an excellent source of beta-carotene, which has been shown to give protection against heart disease, stroke, cataracts and some types of cancer (notably stomach and lung). This is because beta-carotene is a potent eradicator of damaging free radicals. It also assists with vision, in particular night vision.

Like other dried fruit, dried apricots too have great potential to eradicate damaging free radicals – and you probably do not need me to mention the laxative effect

beware the kernel

Don't be tempted to crunch on the stone, because the kernel contains a cyanide compound (laetrile or amygdalin) that can be fatal in large doses, causing respiratory failure, paralysis and, left untreated, ultimately death. Apricot kernels contain small amounts of prussic acid, which is destroyed when heated. There are some safe uses for apricot kernels in apricot brandy and the Italian macaroon-style biscuit cakes known as amaretti di Saronno.

An average serving of 3–4 dried apricots will give you one-third of your daily NSP (fibre) and provide around one-fifth of the RNI for vitamins A and C, plus some iron.

of their NSP (fibre) content. The body can also turn beta-carotene from plant foods such as apricots into vitamin A, which is needed by the immune system and for healthy eyes (most non-vegetarians get enough vitamin A from animal foods).

soft and pleasing

Fresh apricots are also rich in vitamin C, needed for immunity and general health. Despite their soft and pleasing appearance, they also contain a good amount of NSP (fibre). The soluble fibre in apricots is pectin, the type that helps to lower blood cholesterol and through its effects on GI levels helps to provide a steady stream of energy that does not cause sudden rises in blood sugar and demands for insulin. Additionally apricots also contain the sugar alcohol sorbitol, which is absorbed slowly and helps bulk and soften stools – unsurprisingly, this laxative effect is common to other dried fruit as well, prunes are particularly famous for this.

dried fruit differences

Dried apricots are colourful and sweet, making them an excellent snack food and far more nutritious than most mainstream confectionery and biscuit or cake alternatives. They are an even better source of NSP (fibre) than fresh, and are also a rich source of potassium, which is often lacking in a modern diet of processed food. Most Western diets contain too little potassium and too much sodium (table salt). Potassium maintains the sodium balance in cells, helping to prevent high blood pressure. Dried apricots are also one of the richest fruit sources of iron, a mineral lacking in many women's diets, and essential to prevent tiredness, poor immunity and anaemia. The iron from plant foods is not as easily absorbed as from meat. To increase absorption, combine foods like apricots with foods rich in vitamin C, such as citrus juice and fruit, salad and green leafy vegetables.

avoid food additives

Most dried apricots are treated with sulphur dioxide (E220) to preserve and enhance the attractive orange colour, but this preservative can trigger asthma attacks in susceptible people.

However, for the majority of us standard dried and no-need-to-soak or ready to eat dried apricots are fine. Unsulphured apricots are available from health food shops, including the small and unattractive, shrivelled Hunza apricots, eaten by the long-lived people of that region. Incidentally, Hunza longevity has also been attributed to regular consumption of yogurt and the benefits of a healthy gut flora (see page 16) that this engenders.

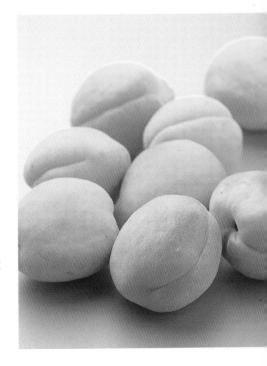

apricot rock buns

These buns will quickly become a family favourite. They have a crisp rocky outside that contrasts with a soft inside containing moist apricot pieces. They also freeze well and are especially delicious eaten warm.

preparation time **15 minutes**
cooking time **15 minutes**
makes **12 small buns**

250 g (8 oz) plain wholemeal flour
1 teaspoon mixed spice
1 teaspoon baking powder
75 g (3 oz) butter or soft vegetable margarine
75 g (3 oz) demerara sugar
125 g (4 oz) dried apricots, chopped
grated rind of ½ a lemon
1 free-range egg
4 tablespoons skimmed milk

1 Lightly oil a baking sheet.
2 Sift the flour, spice and baking powder into a mixing bowl, adding the bran from the sieve.
3 Rub in the fat until the mixture resembles breadcrumbs in consistency. Stir in the sugar, apricots and lemon rind.
4 Beat the egg and milk together and work into the dry ingredients to make a light soft dough. Place forkfuls on to the baking sheet and roughen the surface slightly. Bake in a preheated oven, 220°C (425°F), Gas Mark 7, for 12–15 minutes.
5 Leave the buns to cool. They can be stored in an airtight container for 4–5 days.

spice island apricot strudel

A recipe inspired by the warm, freshly baked, spicy apple strudel in the breakfast baskets of hotels on the spice island of Grenada.

preparation time **15 minutes**
cooking time **20–25 minutes**
serves **8**

500 g (1 lb) canned apricots, drained
1 tablespoon ground cinnamon
2 teaspoons vanilla essence
125 g (4 oz) golden caster sugar
125 g (4 oz) white breadcrumbs
100 g (3½ oz) raisins
200 g (7 oz) filo pastry
25 g (1 oz) butter, melted

1 Lightly oil a baking sheet.
2 Put the apricots, cinnamon, vanilla essence, caster sugar and breadcrumbs into a food processor and blend roughly.
3 Place the pastry sheets in a stack, one on top of the other, brushing with melted butter between each one, and keeping the longer edge facing you.
4 Heap the filling across the longer edge of the pastry, leaving about 5 cm (2 inches) space from the top and sides. Fold the top edge onto the filling and begin rolling up the rest of the pastry, tucking in the edges as you go.
5 Place the strudel on the baking sheet and bake in a preheated oven, 180°C (350°F), Gas Mark 4, for 20–25 minutes or until golden brown. Serve warm with natural yogurt or vanilla ice cream.

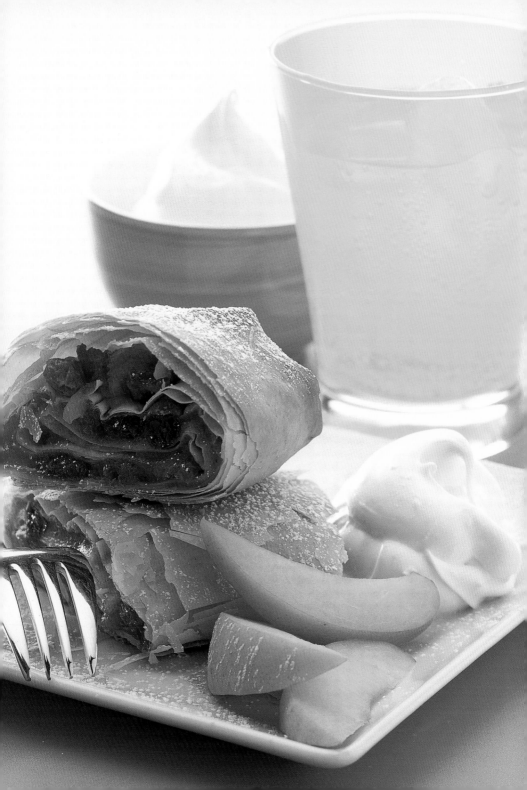

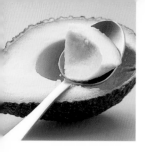

avocados

Avocado is the richest of all fruits, with its high natural oil and protein content. It has long been recognized as a powerful food, having been cultivated in South America for more than 7,000 years. Avocados come in all shapes and sizes from tiny 'cocktail' ones to the gigantic 'family size' fruit.

POWER CONTENT

Vitamin B1, 2 and 6
Vitamin C
Vitamin E
NSP (fibre)
Folates

PLUS POINTS

+ Rich in calories for a useful pre- or post-match salad. Like nuts, its calorie content derives from oils that are mainly unsaturated.

+ Unusually good source of vitamin E for a 'vegetable', protecting against oxidative damage.

+ Also contains B vitamins to assist in healthy nerves.

The Aztecs and Incas knew the value of this pear-shaped fruit, from a member of the laurel tree family, and to them it was an important food. It is also native to Guatemala. It is sometimes called the alligator pear because of its thick, knobbly skin. The main varieties that are widely available are Fuerte, which has a fairly smooth, thin green skin, and Hass, which is smaller with a blackish skin (right).

vitamins and minerals

Avocados are a good source of several vitamins not usually found in vegetables (probably because the avocado is technically a fruit): for example, vitamin E, more commonly found in nuts and vegetable oils; vitamin B6; and folates.

Vitamin E is particularly important for the protection of cell membranes, where it prevents fats being

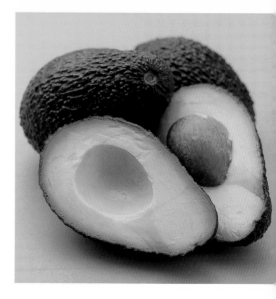

Avocados are useful in the prevention of heart disease, maintaining healthy skin and good circulation.

oxidized and giving rise to harmful free radicals. It also maintains healthy skin, heart and circulation, nerves, muscles and red blood cells. In addition, male fertility can benefit from vitamin E, which plays a role in improving sperm count. The avocado also contains a small amount of B vitamins other than folates, including thiamin (B1) and riboflavin (B2), which are needed for releasing energy. As you might expect for a fruit, it also contains vitamin C.

The mineral copper is found in avocados. Although not much attention is paid to this mineral, it is vital for forming red blood cells and for helping absorb iron from other foods.

nutritious and versatile

Avocados contain a reasonable amount of NSP (fibre) in a very digestible form. In the Caribbean, where the largest varieties grow and they are plentiful, they are mashed to make a spread known as 'poor man's butter' (which is much lower in saturated fat than butter). Blended with yogurt and herbs, avocado can be made into a variety of tasty dips, salad dressings and accompaniments, or just add it in chunks to a salad.

fat as fuel

Up to 30 per cent of an avocado can be oil, making it rich in calories. However, it deserves its healthy reputation because the fats are mainly monounsaturated fats.

Monounsaturates should replace saturated fats in the diet because they reduce harmful types of cholesterol (LDL) without also reducing levels of beneficial HDL cholesterol. In this way, avocados may be a useful food in the prevention of heart disease – although weight-watchers might want to restrict their intake.

Avocados are also a recommended weaning food for babies. They are nutritious, tasty and easy to eat and will mash down to a smooth, digestible purée easily. From four months they can be introduced as a simple purée.

Hard, unripe avocados can be ripened by storing them in a brown paper bag with a banana. Once ripe, they can be stored in the refrigerator for about three more days.

Guacamole

There are many recipes for guacamole in Mexico as each family will have its own variation of this dish, which – eaten on a daily basis in a traditional diet – offers many health benefits. To make a basic guacamole:

1 Halve two ripe avocados, scoop out the flesh and combine with 1–2 crushed garlic cloves and the juice of a lemon or lime.
2 Season to taste with Tabasco sauce, ground cumin and chilli powder.
3 As a variation add finely diced onion and chillies and finely chopped skinned and deseeded tomatoes.

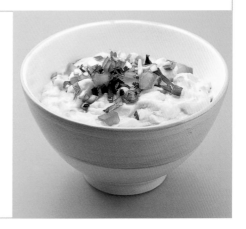

avocado foccaccia

preparation time **2 hours**
cooking time **15 minutes**
makes **2 loaves**

15 g (½ oz) fresh yeast
1 teaspoon sugar
300 ml (½ pint) lukewarm water
200 g (7 oz) plain white or Italian tipo '0' flour
1 tablespoon coarse sea salt, plus 3 pinches
75 ml (3 fl oz) extra virgin olive oil
300 g (10 oz) fine semolina
avocado, bacon, lettuce, tomatoes and vinaigrette
   to fill

1 Oil 2 large baking sheets.
2 Mix the yeast with the sugar and 200 ml (7 fl oz) of
   the water and leave for about 10 minutes, or until it
   starts to almost 'bubble'. Work in the flour with a fork
   and leave for 20 minutes to form a sponge.
3 Dissolve the sponge in the rest of the water, stirring
   well. Add the 3 pinches of salt and 2 tablespoons of
   the olive oil. Mix in the semolina.
4 Turn out on to a work surface and knead the very
   sticky dough for 10 minutes until firm. Put in an oiled
   bowl and leave to rise in a warm place for 1 hour, or
   until doubled in size.
5 Shape the dough straight on to the baking sheets,
   either in 2 thin flat breads about 1 cm (½ inch) thick,
   or 1 large bread about 2.5 cm (1 inch) thick. Make
   indentations all over the top with your fingers.
6 Drizzle over the rest of the olive oil and sprinkle with
   the coarse salt. Leave to rise for 20 minutes, then
   bake in a preheated oven, at 240°C (475°F), Gas
   Mark 9, for 15 minutes, or until crusty and golden.
7 Transfer the bread to a wire rack to cool a little, then,
   while still warm, slice and fill with sliced avocado,
   lettuce, grilled bacon, tomatoes and vinaigrette.

thai avocado & prawn salad

This salad is substantial enough to be a meal in
itself, although if you scale down the quantities you
can also use the recipe as a starter. Lemon may be
used in place of lime, or try half and half.

preparation time **20 minutes**
serves **4**

50 g (2 oz) creamed coconut, grated
2 tablespoons hot water
150 ml (¼ pint) natural yogurt
juice of 1 lime
pinch of chilli powder or cayenne
4 spring onions, chopped
250 g (8 oz) peeled cooked prawns
2 large ripe avocados
1 large crisp lettuce heart
100 g (3½ oz) mustard greens or rocket
1 mango, peeled, pitted and sliced
2 tablespoons whole fresh coriander leaves

1 Mix the coconut and hot water in a bowl and leave
   to cool. Add the yogurt to the bowl with half the lime
   juice and the chilli powder or cayenne.
2 Add the spring onions and prawns.
3 Halve the avocados and discard the stones. Remove
   from the skin by slipping the back of a teaspoon
   between flesh and skin, then gently levering out.
   Slice each half into several thin slices and dress
   with the remaining lime juice.
4 Arrange the lettuce and mustard greens or rocket
   on serving plates. Add the mango slices and
   coriander leaves. Top with the avocado slices and
   spoon over the prawns in their dressing.

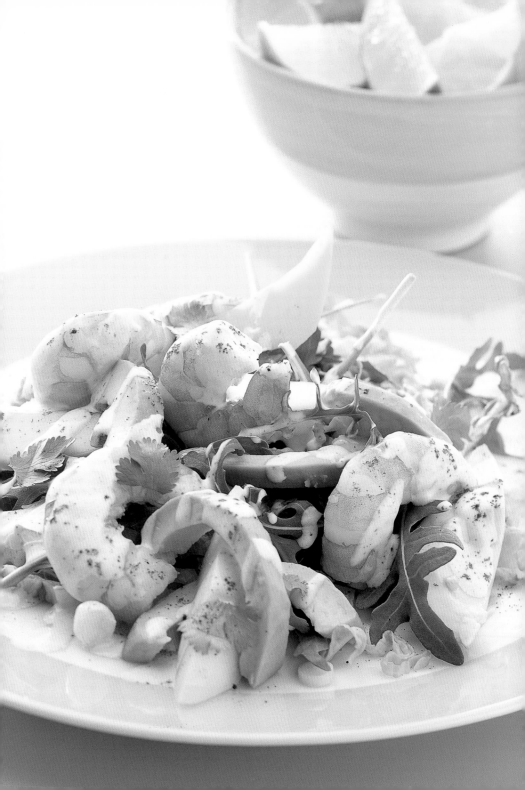

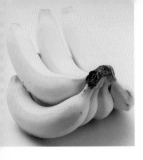

bananas

Popular with everyone from babies to grandparents, bananas are a brilliant food. They power sportspeople through top international events thanks to their concentrated energy, and are also rich in valuable minerals such as potassium. Enjoy alone or add them to breakfast cereals, sandwich fillings and sweet and savoury salads.

POWER CONTENT

Vitamin B6
Vitamin E
NSP (fibre)
Potassium
Natural sugars
GI 55

PLUS POINTS

+ Boosts energy during a round of golf or a tennis game.

+ Have a glass of water and a banana as an alternative to expensive sports drinks for replenishing energy after exhausting activity.

+ Makes a high-energy smoothie drink, which is easier to digest than a bulky snack when you need to eat shortly before doing exercise.

Bananas are packed with slow-release energy, making them better than sugary drinks and confectionery for a quick energy boost. They are unusual among fruit because they are a good source of vitamin B6 and also contribute a small amount of vitamin E. Vitamin B6 (pyridoxine) is important in protein metabolism, and promotes a healthy nervous system and healthy skin. Other B vitamins and minerals in bananas are needed for releasing energy from food during digestion and for maintaining healthy nerves.

a versatile fruit

Bananas need not simply be eaten whole or sliced in a fruit salad. Take advantage of the natural sweetness of ripe bananas and use them mashed, with low-fat soft white cheese to make icing for buns, muffins, cakes (good with carrot cake) and biscuits.

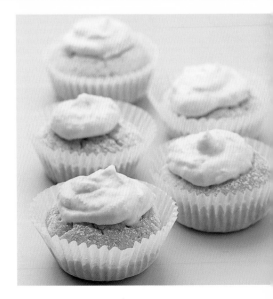

The sugar content of bananas is made up of 7 per cent sucrose, 2 per cent glucose and only 1 per cent fructose. Fructose is fruit sugar and is the sweetest of all the naturally occurring sugars. Glucose is immediately available to the body as it is already in the form of 'blood sugar' and sucrose is – just sugar! It is otherwise known as refined sugar but occurs naturally in this form in some fruit. Bananas are a particularly sweet-tasting fruit and can act as a healthy snack for someone with a sweet tooth. Dried bananas are particularly beneficial used in baking to naturally sweeten dishes; they also have a higher concentration of potassium than the fresh fruit.

ideal weaning food

Bananas are favoured by many people mainly because they are easily digested, which makes them an ideal weaning food. From the age of 4–6 months, a baby is introduced to 'solid' food, and mashed banana is a perfect start. From around 9 months, when 'finger foods' may be offered, babies enjoy eating a slice of banana – it's deliciously soft and suckable and chewy!

health benefits

The NSP (fibre) in bananas feed and maintain a healthy gut flora, encouraging the type of bacteria that boost immunity and aid digestion. Also found in bananas is vitamin B6, which is needed for the formation of infection-fighting antibodies (substances produced in response to body invaders called antigens) and for the formation of haemoglobin in red blood cells. Bananas are also a useful source of potassium that helps to fight age-related rising blood pressure.

power boost

Whatever exercise you have engaged in, whether you have been for a walk, done some gardening or been competing in a sporting event, follow it up with a banana and a drink of water as a healthy way of replenishing energy.

instant energy smoothie

Smoothies are made from fruit juice, or yogurt or milk with added fruit purée. Bananas make a marvellous base ingredient in these drinks, adding sweetness and texture to them. They are versatile and go well with many (ripe) fruits, particularly mango and peaches, and berries such as raspberry or strawberry.

For a drink that is an all-round booster try blending the juice from 150 g (5 oz) of carrot and 100 g (3½ oz) orange with 100 g (3½ oz) of banana and a dried apricot. This smoothie is full of iron, calcium and potassium, which means it is great for bones and teeth as well as for keeping colds at bay.

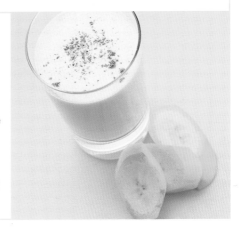

banana muffins

Make these muffins for packed lunches or snacks, or serve with Great Grilled Fruits (see right) as a dessert.

preparation time **20 minutes**
cooking time **20–25 minutes**
makes **10**

200 g (7 oz) plain white organic flour
3 teaspoons baking powder
1½ teaspoons ground cinnamon
grating of fresh nutmeg
50 g (2 oz) ground almonds
50 g (2 oz) soft brown sugar
2 large ripe bananas, about 350 g (11½ oz)
   unpeeled or 250 g (8 oz) peeled
2 free-range eggs
2 tablespoons sunflower oil
125 ml (4 fl oz) skimmed milk
3 tablespoons clear honey

1 Line a muffin tin with 10 paper cases or lightly oil the cups.
2 Sift the flour, baking powder and cinnamon into a bowl. Stir in the nutmeg, almonds and sugar.
3 Lightly mash the banana and work in the eggs, oil, milk and honey to make a sloppy paste. Work the banana mixture into the dry ingredients, first using a fork and then folding in with a tablespoon.
4 Spoon the muffin batter into the paper cases and bake in a preheated oven, 190°C (375°F), Gas Mark 5, for 25 minutes (check after 20 minutes), or until well risen and a skewer inserted in the centre comes out clean.
5 When cold, freeze those muffins that are not to be eaten immediately. To freeze, place in a suitable rigid container with enough headspace not to crush the muffins. Alternatively, place in a freezer bag and extract air from the bag and before sealing. Put the bag or container in the coldest part of the freezer.

great grilled fruits

A hot fruit salad makes a delicious change, and this one is great for summer barbecues because it has that tropical taste. It's good for breakfast at the weekend, too.

preparation time **20 minutes**
cooking time **10–15 minutes**
serves **4**

1 large mango
1 large papaya
2 medium bananas, peeled and halved
2 oranges
25 g (1 oz) butter
40 g (1½ oz) brown sugar
TO SERVE
thick natural yogurt
pancakes (optional)

1 Prepare the fruit. Cut the mango 'cheeks' from the sides of the stone and peel the two halves. Slice or dice the flesh. Halve the papaya and remove the seeds. Peel and slice. Peel the bananas and halve crosswise, then slice the halves in half lengthways. Peel the oranges and slice into circles, removing the pips as you work.
2 Butter a grill pan and arrange the fruit in the pan. Sprinkle over the sugar and place under a very hot grill for 10–15 minutes, turning occasionally and basting with the melted sugar, butter and fruit juices.
3 Serve the fruits with thick natural yogurt and pancakes, if liked.

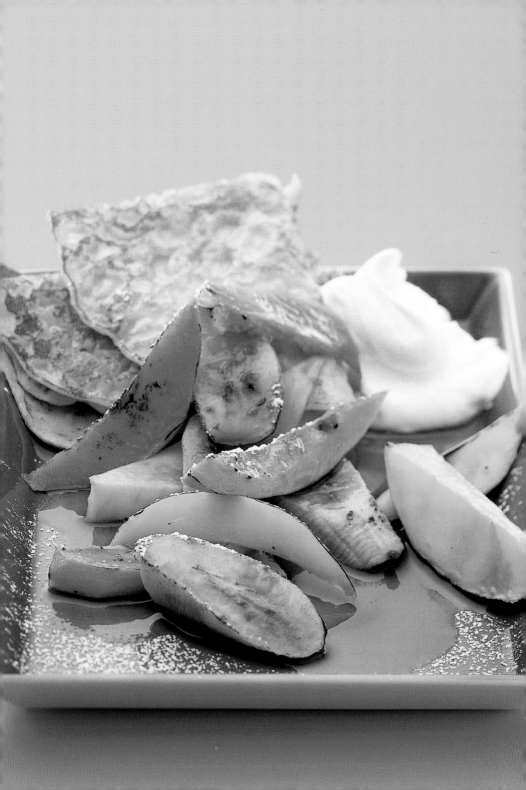

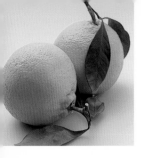

citrus fruit

Oranges are definitely not the only fruit when it comes to citrus – the fruit family known as a rich source of vitamin C. Other foods may be richer in this vitamin (blackcurrants, guavas and green peppers), but none is so universally accessible and popular as citrus in all its varieties: grapefruit, lemons, limes, and easy-peelers like clementines and satsumas.

POWER CONTENT

Vitamin C
NSP (fibre)
Iron
Potassium
Sorbitol
Beta-carotene
GI 57 (fresh)
GI 31 (dried)

PLUS POINTS

+ Wedges of oranges should never have been abandoned as a half-time refresher for footballers because they provide a boost of antioxidant and immune-enhancing vitamin C.

+ Good source of folic acid for the production of red blood cells to carry oxygen, needed for turning food into energy for sports.

+ Rich in rutin, a flavonoid that has an anti-inflammatory effect and so helps to heal bumps and knocks associated with physical activity.

Vitamin C is perhaps the best-known vitamin, being one of the first to be discovered and one that has such obvious and immediate effects; with a deficiency resulting in scurvy. Ever since limes and lemons were given to sailors on long voyages to prevent them from developing the disease, citrus fruit has been linked to good health.

More recently, we have improved our understanding of vitamin C's role in boosting immunity. It is an antioxidant and therefore able to neutralize potentially damaging free radicals. Vitamin C's function in the immune system is to help the white blood cells fight infection and it is essential for wound-healing.

Vitamin C is also needed for the formation of collagen and connective tissue, in the skin, nails and hair, and for the formation of bones, teeth and capillaries.

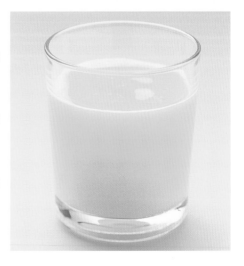

citrus strengths

It surprises many people to learn that oranges also supply a reasonable amount of folates. Essential for brain and spinal cord development during the earliest weeks of pregnancy they help to reduce the risk of the devastating birth defect spina bifida. Adequate folates also reduce the risk of heart disease by lowering blood levels of the amino acid homocysteine (see page 13). In addition, folic acid is essential for the formation of red blood cells to prevent anaemia and tiredness.

Oranges and orange juice are on a par with cooked soya beans, cauliflower, cooked chickpeas, potatoes, iceberg lettuce and peas in the amount of folates that they contain.

A group of antioxidants called flavonoids are also found in citrus fruit. They work with vitamin C to boost immunity and strengthen blood capillaries, and they also have an anti-inflammatory effect. One flavonoid called rutin, found in citrus (and blackcurrants), helps protect blood capillaries that prevent or heal broken veins. Another flavonoid called limonoid increases the production of enzymes that help the body dispose of carcinogens.

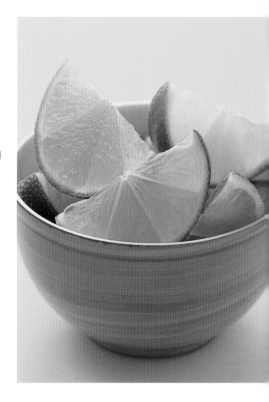

A daily glass of orange or grapefruit juice reduces the risk of stroke.

marmalade can be good for you!

The flavonoids found in citrus fruit survive high temperatures when being made into marmalade, as do the antioxidants, terpenes and liminoids that help strengthen blood capillaries and enhance the effects of vitamin C. Pectin, the gummy soluble fibre in citrus fruit which sets marmalade (and other preserves), has cholesterol-lowering abilities in its raw state in fresh fruit. However, marmalade should not be eaten in quantities large enough to make a notable contribution of NSP (fibre) to the diet because it is a sugary food.

citrus tips

One medium-to-large orange provides 80 mg of vitamin C, twice the RNI for all adults.

Although orange and other citrus juices are tremendously healthy, alone they cannot provide the 5 portions of fruit and vegetables needed each day for health. This is because many of the phytochemicals attached to the 'body' of the fruit and vegetables (e.g. rutin in the pith, see Plus Points, left) are removed when making juice.

marmalade gammon steaks

Gammon steaks are quick and easy to prepare, and the bacon flavour goes well with citrus, which combats the saltiness and refreshes the palate.

preparation time **10 minutes**
cooking time **25 minutes**
serves **4**

4 gammon steaks
4 tablespoons redcurrant jelly
juice of 2 oranges and 1 large lemon
3 tablespoons fine-cut marmalade,
    preferably home-made

1 Remove the rind from the gammon and slash the fatty edges to avoid the steaks curling.
2 Place the steaks in a shallow ovenproof dish. Spread the top of each steak with redcurrant jelly.
3 Mix the citrus juice with the marmalade and pour over the gammon, making sure the shreds of peel land on the gammon.
4 Cook in a preheated oven, 180°C (350°F), Gas Mark 4, for about 25 minutes, or until the gammon is browned but not dried out on the surface. Remove the steaks from the dish and cut off any excess fat. Serve on warmed plates. Spoon a little of the sauce over each steak, and pour the rest into a small jug to serve separately. Serve with a green vegetable and some mashed potato.

pink grapefruit & pine nut salad

A refreshing, light salad that can be served with a jacket potato or bread to make a more filling meal.

preparation time **15 minutes**
cooking time **3–4 minutes**
serves **4**

2 pink grapefruit, peeled and segmented
2 avocados, stones removed, peeled and sliced
75 g (3 oz) pine nuts
200 g (7 oz) baby spinach leaves or lamb's lettuce
1 Romaine lettuce head, leaves washed and dried
4 tablespoons grated Parmesan cheese
FOR THE DRESSING
3 tablespoons sunflower, corn or other light
    vegetable oil
2 teaspoons white wine vinegar
1 teaspoon smooth mustard, such as Dijon
sea salt and freshly ground black pepper

1 Prepare the grapefruit, working over a dish to reserve the juice.
2 Prepare the avocados, and mix with the reserved citrus juice to prevent the flesh discolouring.
3 Lightly toast the pine nuts under a grill or dry-fry in a frying pan.
4 Place all the dressing ingredients in a clean screw-top jar and shake vigorously or whisk in a jug. Toss the prepared leaves in the dressing, then arrange on 4 individual plates or in salad bowls.
5 Arrange the avocado and grapefruit over the leaves. Sprinkle over the pine nuts and offer the Parmesan separately at the table.

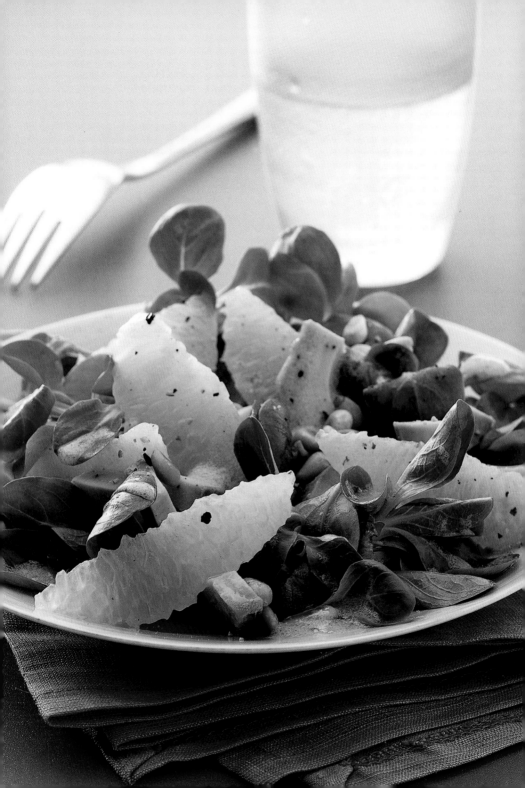

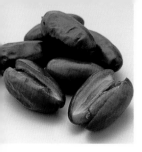

dates

Like bananas, dates are a great energy food for snacks and for use by sportspeople when training and recovering from exhausting activities. They are sweet and satsifying while also being packed with nutrients and fibre.

POWER CONTENT
Vitamin B3 and 6
NSP (fibre)
Iron
Magnesium
Potassium
Beta-carotene

PLUS POINTS
+ One of the most concentrated 'sugary' fruits available for a pre- or post-sports snack.

+ The fibre content moderates the speed at which energy is released, making them better than sweets and confectionery.

+ Contains minerals that make up antioxidant enzymes to protect against exercise-induced free-radical damage.

Dates are a staple food in the Arab world, but until recently they were available only in dried form, either whole as a Christmas treat or as a compressed block for cooking. Now, however, sophisticated frozen and chilled transport means that fresh dates are a permanent 'luxury' in our supermarkets and grocery outlets. Fresh dates are frozen for export from Egypt, Iraq, Iran, Israel and North Africa. The fresh dates we buy in punnets are defrosted, but the process has a minimal effect on their texture and flavour, as their high sugar content protects them.

Many varieties of dates are familiar throughout the Arab world, but only a few of the semi-dry varieties sold as fresh dates are available to us. The most common are Deglet Noor and Halawi, although the variety is not always stated on the packs. Medjool, a deep red date with thick flesh and little fibre, is becoming more popular.

sweet and nutritious
In both their fresh and dried form, dates are one of the most convenient snack foods. They have all the sweet attractions of confectionery, and although they are 'sugary' and a good source of energy, they also contain

date purée

Date purée is an excellent substitute for some or all of the fat in a recipe when baking. Obviously, the finished item will be different, and you will need to experiment with recipes. To make date purée, simmer dried dates in enough water to prevent them sticking to the bottom of the pan and burning. When soft, beat to a purée with a wooden spoon.

nutrients. They are rich in NSP (fibre) and some people find them a gentle form of laxative.

Dates contain beta-carotene, vitamin B6 and niacin (B3). They are also rich in the mineral potassium, needed for maintaining the sodium balance in cells and helping to prevent high blood pressure. Other minerals found in dates include magnesium, iron and copper. Fresh dates contain some vitamin C, but their main benefit is as a high energy fruit.

enjoying dates

Fresh dates can be eaten just as they are, without having to remove the thin, papery skin. On the Medjool date the skin is so soft and integral that it would in fact be impossible to remove. After removing the central stone, dates may also be stuffed with a filling, such as low-fat soft cheese.

Dried dates can also be eaten as they are, or can be chopped and used in cakes, scones, muffins or mixed into breakfast cereal or fruit salads.

a date with the dentist

While dates are a more nutritious form of sugary energy than confectionery, they do have potential dental health drawbacks. The more frequently you consume sugary foods and drinks, the greater your risk of dental decay – hence the advice to eat confectionery as part of a meal, if at all. Sugary drinks that are slowly sipped have the same effect, and acid drinks such as colas and other fizzy drinks are even worse, because the acid attacks the enamel of the teeth; this kind of decay is far more difficult for the dentist to fix than caries. So drink these products only occasionally, or only with meals as this will reduce the number of times they can attack your teeth.

removing stones

Date stones are inedible. To remove the central stone split open the date lengthways and ease out the stone using the point of a sharp knife if it does not come out easily.

Medjool dates

Medjool dates, primarily from Israel, should be plump, but they do not have the smooth shiny skins of normal dates because they are a different variety and their skins are naturally wrinkled with a matt finish. You are unlikely to see Medjool dates in poor condition, because they are luxury goods and are usually sold in small protective plastic punnets of around 200 g (7 oz), containing ten 20 g (¾ oz) dates.

Store them in a cool dry place if they are to be eaten within a week, or in the refrigerator where they can be stored for up to 1 month.

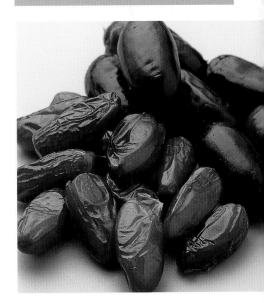

date & walnut cake

A tasty sponge using a blend of wholemeal and white flour for extra fibre. The nuts and dates also add fibre, plus vitamins and, most importantly, a winning flavour combination.

preparation time **20 minutes**
cooking time **25–30 minutes**
makes **8–10 slices**

125g (4 oz) butter
125g (4 oz) golden caster or soft brown sugar
2 free-range eggs
75 g (3 oz) self-raising white organic flour, sifted
50 g (2 oz) plain wholemeal organic flour
60 g (2½ oz) dried dates, chopped
60 g (2½ oz) walnuts, chopped

1 Lightly oil a 1 kg (2 lb) loaf tin.
2 Cream the butter and sugar together until pale and creamy, with a soft dropping consistency.
3 Lightly beat in the eggs, adding a little white flour between additions if the mixture starts to curdle.
4 Fold in the remaining flour, dates and walnuts and spoon the mixture into the prepared tin. Place in a preheated oven, 180°C (350°F), Gas Mark 4, for 25–30 minutes, or until a skewer inserted in the centre comes out clean.
5 Turn out of the tin while warm and leave to cool on a rack before serving.

date flapjacks

Most people love flapjacks and these are extra special as they have a lovely moist and gooey centre.

preparation time **12 minutes**
cooking time **18–20 minutes**
makes **12 small flapjacks**

300 g (10 oz) dates, stoned
100 ml (3½ fl oz) water
75 g (3 oz) butter or margarine
125 g (4 oz) demerara sugar
1 tablespoon golden syrup
300 g (10 oz) porridge oats

1 Lightly oil an 18 cm (7 inch) square cake tin, preferably loose-bottomed.
2 Put the dates and water in a saucepan with a well-fitting lid and cook over a low heat for 10 minutes, occasionally breaking up the dates using the back of a wooden spoon until they are pulpy. Remove and blend to a thick purée in a food processor.
3 Melt the butter, sugar and golden syrup in a saucepan over a moderate heat, stirring to dissolve the sugar. Remove from the heat.
4 Put the oats in a bowl and stir in the melted butter mixture. Lightly press half the oat mixture into the base of the prepared tin. Spread the date mixture over the top. Cover with the remaining oats and press down lightly.
5 Place in a preheated oven, 180°C (350°F), Gas Mark 4, for 18–20 minutes, or until golden brown. Remove from the oven and put the tin on a wire rack. Cut through into squares while the flapjacks are hot, but leave to set in the tin until completely cold. Slice the flapjacks again and remove from the tin.

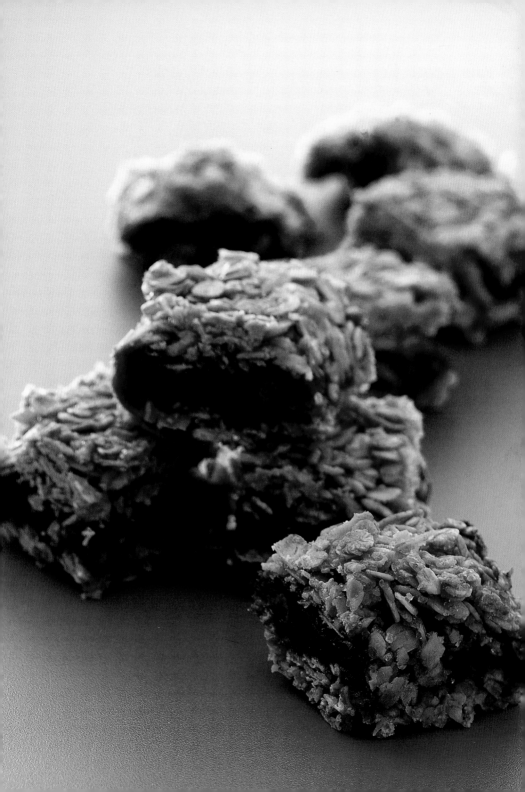

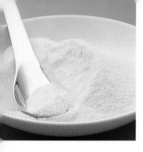

corn

North American Indians and Aztecs relied on corn and beans as their staple foods. The corn breads of the Aztec and Maya, tortillas and tamales, are still a staple in Mexico and are now known internationally. Corn chips for dipping into salsas have brought new popularity to this food – and even blue corn varieties are now available.

POWER CONTENT
Vitamin B1 and B3
NSP (fibre)
Iron
Carotenoids
Folates
GI 55 (canned sweetcorn)
GI 68 (polenta)

PLUS POINTS
+ Good source of the eye-protective carotenoids essential for outdoor sportspeople from walkers to marathon-runners.

+ Excellent source of fibre for slow-release energy that does not disrupt blood-sugar levels.

+ Versatile carbohydrate food, particularly useful for those who cannot tolerate wheat or other starchy staples.

Corn is probably better known to Europeans as sweetcorn. The kernels of corn-on-the-cob rose in popularity as a vegetable in the UK after being imported from the United States. The use of ground cornmeal by our nearer neighbours, the Italians, to make polenta has never really caught on widely in the rest of Europe, although this hitherto Italian peasant food can now be found on the menu in some restaurants.

versatility of corn
Ground corn, called cornmeal, is commonly used in the southern states of America to make soft breads, often enriched with eggs and butter. Cornbread is, like cake-type tea breads, risen by the addition of baking agents such as baking powder, or a combination of bicarbonate of soda and cream of tartar. But cornbreads have not

become an everyday staple elsewhere. The breakfast cereal cornflakes, in contrast is eaten around the world. Although a nutritious cereal, it is high in salt, so eat only occasionally and avoid it if you have high blood pressure.

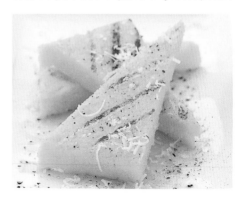

fibre provider

Maize, or corn, is an excellent source of NSP (fibre). Anyone who has eaten and enjoyed corn-on-the-cob can testify to the amount of fibre that is left between their teeth. NSP has been associated with lower cholesterol levels.

An average cob provides about one-third of your daily NSP needs. The canned equivalent – 85 g (just over 3 oz) of sweetcorn kernels – provides just under one-quarter. Sweetcorn, like carrots and peas, has a low glycaemic index (see page 8). This means they release energy slowly and do not disrupt blood sugar levels, keeping you on an even keel and helping to prevent maturity-onset diabetes. However, when ground to a meal for baking or making into polenta, corn contains very little NSP, because the outer hull has been removed and only the hard part of the endosperm in the middle is used. The soft part is milled into the familiar thickener cornflour.

releasing the goodness

Like other cereals, maize is only a moderate source of protein, but then it is not eaten for its protein content – unless in combination with other vegetable sources, such as the ancient Inca diet of maize, corn breads and beans. Maize contains fewer B vitamins than other cereals, and the niacin (B3) is in a form that is biologically unavailable until the maize has been treated with heat and an alkaline solution. In Central America, where maize is the main source of energy, it is treated with lime water to release the niacin. The process also adds calcium to the corn. Corn is unusual among grains in that it contains carotenoids (types of carotene), in particular the antioxidants lutein and zeaxanthin. Other good sources are red peppers, peas, celery and cooked tomatoes.

perfect polenta

Polenta is made by grinding maize to a meal. It is not rich in protein, but its benefits include the fact that it is gluten-free and contains useful amounts of thiamin (B1) and iron, plus some niacin (B3) and protein.

Polenta meal can be coarse or fine. Both types are simmered and boiled with water to make a thick paste that can be served as an alternative to rice or potatoes. The paste may also be put in an oiled baking tin, baked in the oven, then cut into slices and eaten hot or cold or grilled. Grated cheese, especially Parmesan, can be added to the mixture (polenta is rather bland), or slices of cheese can be grilled on top of polenta.

Polenta is traditionally added to boiling water, but this can lead to a lumpy paste. To avoid this, add it to cold water and bring it to the boil.

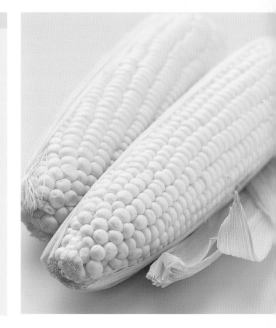

welsh rarebit cornbread

Susanne Beard, a friend and keen cook, devised this power food recipe for her teenage sons. As an alternative, substitute the cheese with 75 g (3 oz) of chopped chorizo sausage.

preparation time **15 minutes**
cooking time **20–25 minutes**
makes **8 slices**

125 g (4 oz) cornmeal or polenta
125 g (4 oz) plain flour
2 rounded teaspoons baking powder
½ teaspoon English mustard powder
200 g (7 oz) can sweetcorn kernels, drained
150 g (5 oz) strong mature Cheddar cheese,
    coarsely grated
1 large free-range egg, lightly beaten
200 ml (7 fl oz) skimmed milk
2 tablespoons olive oil
½ teaspoon Worcestershire sauce
generous amount of salt, freshly ground black
    pepper and freshly grated nutmeg, to taste

1 Line a 500 g (1 lb) loaf tin with baking parchment.
2 Put the cornmeal or polenta, flour, baking powder and mustard in a mixing bowl and season with salt, pepper and nutmeg.
3 Stir in the sweetcorn and cheese.
4 Lightly beat the egg, milk, olive oil and Worcestershire sauce. Add to the bowl and mix in with a fork.
5 Pour the mixture into the prepared tin and bake in a preheated oven, 220°C (425°F), Gas Mark 7, for 20–25 minutes until golden and slightly crusty, or an inserted skewer comes out clean.
6 Cool in the tin for 5 minutes, then turn out on to a plate. Serve warm or cold, with salad or vegetables.

polenta with chicken & chilli relish

preparation time **25 minutes**
cooking time **50 minutes**
serves **4**

150 g (5 oz) quick-cook polenta or cornmeal
250 ml (8 fl oz) cold water
450 ml (¾ pint) chicken stock
2 tablespoons extra virgin olive oil
4 chicken drumsticks
1 large onion
2 garlic cloves, diced
2 fresh red chillies, deseeded and diced
½ butternut (or similar) squash, about 400 g
    (13 oz), cut into strips
400 g (13 oz) can tomatoes
1 bay leaf

1 Blend the polenta or cornmeal with the water in a bowl. Bring the stock to the boil in a saucepan and add the polenta mixture in one go. Stir over a moderate heat until the mixture boils and thickens. Reduce the heat and simmer for 5 minutes, or until very thick. Serve either 'wet' as it is now, or remove the pan from the heat and spoon the mixture into an oiled 20 cm (8 inch) tin. Smooth the top and leave until completely cold, then cut into squares or wedges. To serve, lightly brush with olive oil and fry or grill for 3 minutes either side until golden.
2 Heat the oil in a casserole over the hob and add the chicken, onion, garlic, chillies and squash. Cover and cook for 10 minutes.
3 Stir in the tomatoes and bay leaf and transfer to a preheated oven, 180°C (350°F), Gas Mark 4, for 40 minutes.
4 Serve with the polenta in the style of your choice and with green vegetables if liked.

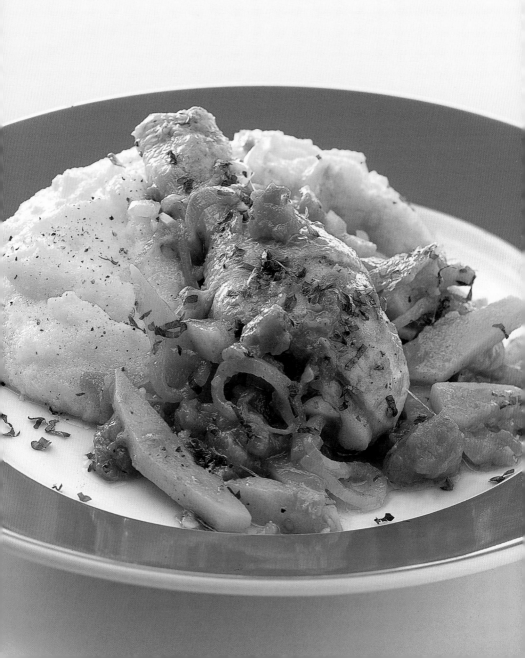

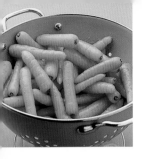

carrots

It's true, carrots can help you see in the dark, because they are a good source of beta-carotene and other types of carotene that are turned into vitamin A, which is essential for night vision.

POWER CONTENT

Vitamin C
Vitamin E
NSP (fibre)
Beta-carotene
Alpha-lipoic acid
GI 49 (peeled and boiled)

PLUS POINTS

+ Rich source of antioxidant vitamins that protect against potential free radical damage caused by aerobic activity.

+ Important source of carotenoids that protect the eyes from ultra-violet damage – useful for outdoor sports enthusiasts.

+ Contains a key component for the conversion of food to energy.

Carrots are good news for everyone who is using power foods to stay younger and fitter for longer, because two types of carotene in carrots – lutein and zeaxanthin – may help to prevent ultra-violet light damaging the lens of the eye, thus reducing the risk of age-related cataracts.

Studies show that people who eat carrots regularly also have a reduced risk of cancers of the lungs, stomach, bladder and other sites.

more powerful than most

Carrots contain a very powerful antioxidant enzyme called alpha-lipoic acid that can reinvigorate the antioxidant vitamins A, C and E, allowing them to repeatedly quench free radicals. Alpha-lipoic acid is also an antioxidant in its own right. It is made naturally in the body and has an important role in the Krebs cycle (the chemical conversion of food to energy). Its small chemical structure allows it to

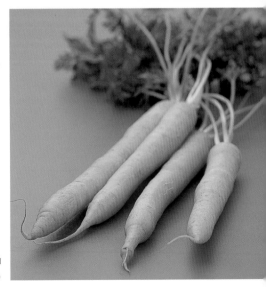

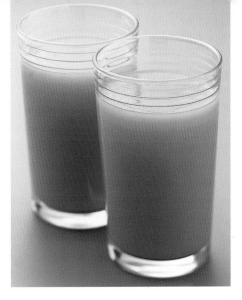

slimming power

Drinking a couple of glasses of water before a meal is an old slimming trick to help fill you up so that you have less room for food and so take in fewer calories. Try a glass of carrot juice instead – it may have calories, but it's great for health. Eating foods with a high water content, such as carrot soup, also reduces the calorie content of the meal. The recipe on page 50 has the added bonus of being very nutritious.

pass through cell membranes that other antioxidants cannot get through, therefore offering protection inside cells as well as outside. It is also found in significant quantities in potatoes (see page 60).

are organic carrots better?

Organic carrots are among the best-selling organic vegetables in supermarkets. They are an important staple for families with babies (carrots are an excellent weaning food) and young children (because they are sweet, carrots are many children's preferred vegetable).

Studies on nutritional content and flavour of organic versus non-organic produce have mixed results and are not particularly conclusive. Wash or scrub all produce thoroughly before use, even if it is organic.

pesticide perils

The popularity of organic carrots is probably also linked to the fact that a government warning is in force in the UK on non-organic carrots. They advise that non-organic carrots should be topped, tailed and peeled to remove pesticide concentrations, especially when fed to babies, toddlers and young children. Some vegetables are more affected by pesticide and other agrochemcial residues than others. Routine government tests show the highest residue levels are usually found in lettuce, spinach and carrots; and for fruit, in pears, apples and apple juice.

can carrots reduce the risk of cancer?

Trials to see whether smokers were less at risk of lung cancer if they took beta-carotene supplements were halted when it was realized that there was actually an increase in risk. Similarly, taking carotene every other day for 12 years did not protect male doctors who were taking part in a physicians' health study against non-melanoma skin cancer, even though it had been shown to protect laboratory mice. However, eating beta-carotene when it is a natural part of foods such as carrots has been shown to be protective against lung and other cancers.

GI goodness

Carrots, sweetcorn (see page 44) and peas (see page 52) share the distinction of having a low glycaemic index (GI, see page 8). This means they release energy slowly and do not disrupt blood-sugar levels, keeping you on an even keel and helping prevent maturity-onset diabetes.

Beta-carotene (pro-vitamin A) is found in orange, red, yellow and dark green vegetables and fruit. Carrots are an excellent source, along with spinach and broccoli, apricots, melon, pumpkin and other squash varieties.

carrot & coriander soup

A wonderful lunch or supper dish – serve with crusty wholegrain bread and make it as smooth or as chunky as you like. One of my recipe tasters was very impressed with the power of this carrot soup – she was shattered before she had it for lunch, but felt her energy return by the mouthful.

preparation time **15 minutes**
cooking time **25 minutes**
serves **4**

60 g (2½ oz) split red lentils
2 tablespoons olive oil
1 onion, chopped
1 large potato, cubed
375 g (12 oz) carrots, peeled and cubed
900 ml (1½ pints) vegetable stock
15 g (½ oz) coriander leaves, chopped
grating of fresh nutmeg (optional)
salt and freshly ground black pepper

1 Rinse the lentils and check for debris. Cover with boiling water and leave for 10 minutes while you prepare the vegetables.
2 Heat the oil in a large heavy-bottomed pan, and sauté the onion for 5 minutes to soften.
3 Add the potato, carrots, lentils in their soaking water and stock. Bring to the boil, lower the heat and simmer for 20 minutes, or until everything is very soft.
4 Transfer to a blender or processor, or blend with a stick blender in the pan to the desired consistency.
5 When ready to serve, reheat the soup very gently if necessary. Check the seasoning, and add fresh coriander and a little grated nutmeg, if liked.

gingered-up carrot cake

preparation time **30 minutes**
cooking time **40–45 minutes**
serves **8**

50 g (2 oz) butter or margarine
25 g (1 oz) soft brown sugar
125 g (4 oz) date purée (see page 40)
2 eggs, lightly beaten
150 g (5 oz) grated carrot
2 pieces of stem ginger, finely chopped
175 g (6 oz) wholemeal flour
2 teaspoons baking powder
1 teaspoon ground cinnamon
25 g (1 oz) golden flax seeds
125 ml (4 fl oz) milk
FOR THE FROSTING
50 g (2 oz) softened butter
100 g (3½ oz) sifted icing sugar
2 tablespoons orange juice
grated rind of ½ an orange
2–3 drops of orange flower water (optional)
candied peel to decorate (optional)

1 Line the base of a 22 cm (8½ inch) cake tin with parchment. Cream the butter and sugar until soft. Work in the date purée. Lightly beat in the eggs, then stir in the carrot and ginger.
2 Sift the flour, baking powder and cinnamon and stir in the seeds. Fold the dry ingredients into the creamed mixture, adding milk as you work to soften the mixture.
3 Spoon into the prepared tin and level the top. Place in a preheated oven, 180°C (350°F), Gas Mark 4, and bake for 40–45 minutes, or until a skewer comes out clean. Cover the top with baking parchment for the last 15 minutes if it is becoming too brown.
4 To make the frosting, beat all the ingredients together until soft. When the cake is completely cold, cover with frosting.

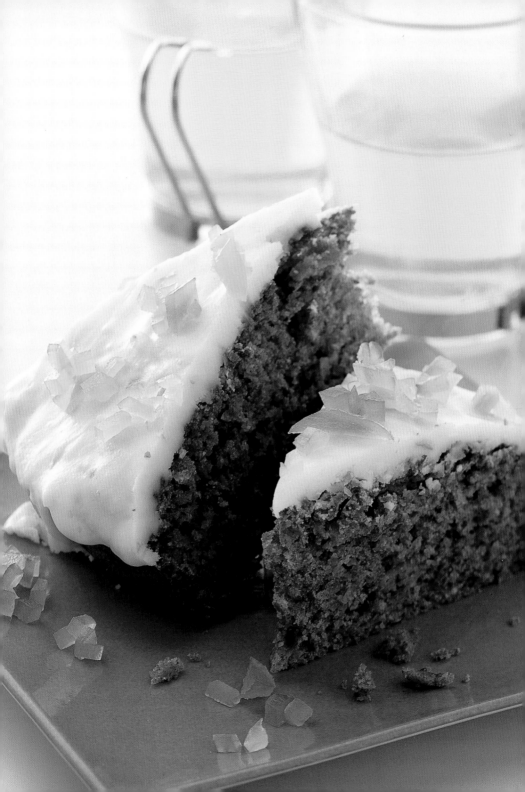

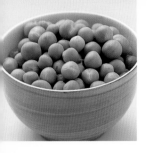

peas

Picked and eaten fresh from the garden, green peas taste wonderful, while frozen peas must be among the world's most nutritious, and still very tasty, convenience foods. Peas belong to the legume family and, along with beans and other pulses, are a valuable and underrated source of vegetarian protein.

POWER CONTENT

B vitamins
Vitamin C
Iron
Protein
Zinc
Carotene
Folates
GI 48 (fresh, boiled), GI 22 (dried, boiled)

PLUS POINTS

+ Richer in protein than many vegetables, making them valuable for vegetarian sports enthusiasts.

+ Contain eye-protective carotenoids essential for those pursuing outdoor activities.

+ Good source of vitamin C, which can be lost as a result of sustained physical activity.

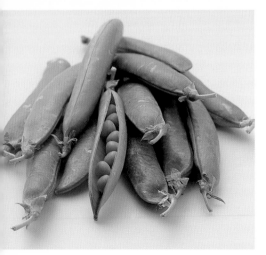

Peas are one of the oldest vegetables known to Western man. Their origins have been traced back some 5,000 years to the lands around the Eastern Mediterranean. Peas have long been one of the most popular vegetables because of their sweet-tasting freshness, and it is possibly this familiarity that has led people to overlook their many nutritional benefits.

nutrition

Peas are a good source of protein. During the Middle Ages, the poor were largely sustained by pease pottage, a thick vegetable soup made with dried peas; peas were not eaten fresh until the fifteenth century.

An average 70 g (just under 3 oz) portion of peas provides nearly half an adult's daily recommended

Eating or drinking vitamin C-rich foods and drinks (such as orange juice, for example) at the same meal as peas will help improve the intake of vegetable iron.

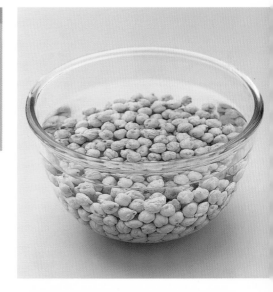

full of folates

Like peas, chickpeas are rich in folate. They are also a good source of carbohydrate, vegetarian protein and dietary fibre. They also contain plant hormones called lignans (see page 73 and 101), which are thought to protect against heart disease, osteoporosis and menopausal problems in women.

nutrient intake (RNI) of vitamin C. Peas also contain the carotenes lutein and zeathanin, which may help prevent ultra-violet light damaging the lens of the eye, and the development of cataracts. Unusually for a vegetable, peas are full of B vitamins, in particular thiamin, needed for transmitting messages between the brain and the spinal cord and for enzymes that convert food into fuel for the body. Women in the early stages of pregnancy should note that peas contain folates, which help prevent the development of spina bifida in the unborn child. The list of their other benefits is long: peas also contain, for a vegetable, a fair amount of iron, protective against anaemia, and zinc, which is good for male fertility; howeve, the iron and zinc found in meat and fish are more easily absorbed by the body.

fresh vs frozen peas

Without wishing to denigrate fresh peas, it is worth remembering that frozen peas can be a better source of vitamin C. This is because large-scale producers can freeze their peas within a few hours of harvesting, whereas fresh peas may take some days to reach the greengrocer and then a few more may elapse before they are purchased, cooked and eaten. Very fresh young peas (petits pois) can be eaten raw, an added bonus, for further vitamins are lost when peas are boiled before eating.

peas take on cholesterol

Peas can help in the battle to lower cholesterol levels, together with other vegetables and fruit such as corn, garlic, onions, haricot beans, apples and pears.

Along with carrots and sweetcorn, fresh and frozen peas share the distinction of having a low glycaemic index. This means they release energy slowly into the bloodstream and do not disrupt blood sugar levels, keeping you on an even keel and helping prevent the onset of diabetes.

taking the pulse

Substituting some meat or meat products or extending meat dishes with pulses, nuts or seeds is beneficial for everyone. Vegetarians in particular are recommended to eat at least 30g (1oz) per day. Pulses are fantastically versatile, low in fat and high in protein and fibre.

vegetable samosas

preparation time **45 minutes**
cooking time **15 minutes**
makes **about 20 (can be frozen)**

2 tablespoons vegetable oil
1 garlic clove, crushed
1 fresh red chilli, deseeded and diced
1 cm (½ inch) fresh root ginger, grated
1 teaspoon ground cumin
2 teaspoons black mustard seeds
1 small sweet potato, peeled and diced
½ a pepper, cored, deseeded and diced
1 small onion, diced
150 g (5 oz) peas, fresh or frozen
1 tablespoon chopped fresh coriander
200 g (7 oz) filo pastry
25 g (1 oz) butter, melted

1 Grease 2 or 3 baking sheets.
2 Heat the oil in a heavy-based pan and sauté the
  garlic, chilli, ginger, cumin, mustard seeds, sweet
  potato, pepper and onion in the oil for 10 minutes,
  stirring occasionally to prevent the mixture sticking.
3 Add the peas, cover with a lid and continue to cook
  over a low heat for 5 minutes, stirring occasionally.
4 Remove from the heat and stir in the coriander.
  Spread the filling on to a shallow dish or tray to cool.
5 Cut the filo sheets in half lengthways. Stack and
  keep covered with a damp teatowel while you work,
  to prevent the pastry from drying out.
6 Brush around the edge of each sheet with melted
  butter. Put a spoonful of filling about 1 cm (½ inch)
  thick in the centre of the pastry and fold over into
  a triangle around the filling. Brush the top and base
  with more melted butter and put on a baking sheet.
  Prepare the rest of the samosas in the same way.
7 Place the sheets in a preheated oven, 190°C
  (375°F), Gas Mark 5, for about 12 minutes, or until
  golden brown. Serve hot or cold.

summer green pea soup

Fabulous with fresh peas, but because of the high
quality of frozen peas this recipe can be enjoyed
all year round.

preparation time **10 minutes or longer if shelling
fresh peas**
cooking time **about 15 minutes**
serves **4**

1 bunch spring onions
1 tablespoon butter
1.25 kg (2½ lb) fresh peas, shelled, or 500 g (1 lb)
    frozen peas
750 ml (1¼ pints) vegetable stock
2 tablespoons thick natural yogurt or single cream
nutmeg
1 tablespoon chopped chives, to garnish

1 Trim, wash and chop the spring onions. Melt the
  butter in a large pan and soften the onions, but
  do not allow them to colour.
2 Add the peas to the pan with the stock. Bring to
  the boil and simmer for about 5 minutes for frozen
  peas, but for up to 15 minutes for fresh peas, until
  they are cooked. Be careful not to overcook fresh
  peas or you will lose the flavour.
3 Remove from the heat and liquidize or pass through
  a mouli vegetable mill.
4 Add the yogurt or cream and grate in a little nutmeg.
  Reheat the soup gently if necessary, and serve
  sprinkled with chives.

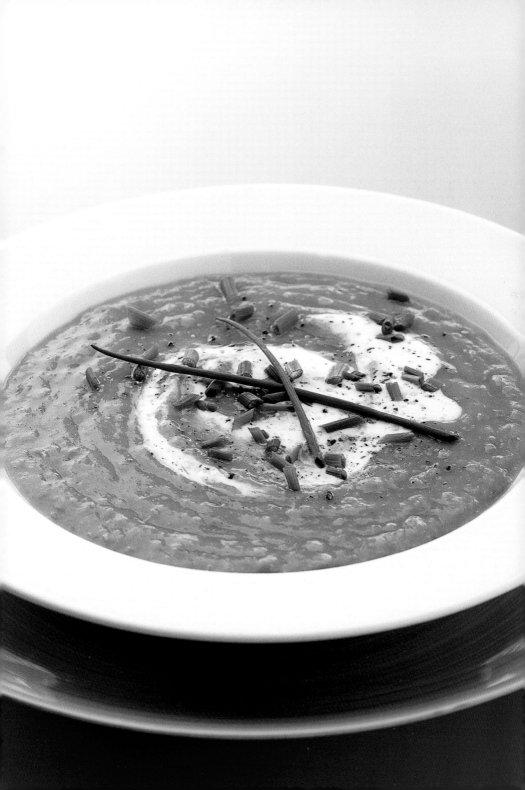

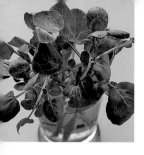

watercress

Those who enjoy the spicy taste of this luxuriously foliaged salad plant will not be surprised to learn that it is related to the mustard plant. The ancient Greeks were aware of its benefits and soldiers ate it as a tonic.

POWER CONTENT

Vitamin C
NSP (fibre)
Iron
Potassium
Sorbitol
Beta-carotene
GI 57 (fresh)

PLUS POINTS

+ Good source of B vitamins and some vitamin E to protect the nerves and heart from sporting wear and tear.

+ Superb combination of carotene and iron for boosting the blood in its oxygen-delivery system.

+ The carotenoids offer particular protection to the eyes from ultra-violet light, so good for outdoor sportspeople.

gloriously green

Watercress owes some of the colour in its luxuriously deep green and glossy foliage to its high level of beta-carotene and iron. Unlike orange vegetables and fruit, the characteristic carotenoid colours are masked in watercress by chlorophyll, the green pigment that allows plants to photosynthesize (make energy from sunlight).

In particular, watercress is a good source of the carotenoids lutein and zeaxanthin, which help prevent degenerative eye diseases such as age-related macular degeneration and cataracts. The macular is the centre of the retina that distinguishes fine detail at the centre of your field of vision. Lutein and zeaxanthin are the only carotenoids found in the lens of the eye and in the macular. Higher than average intake of lutein and zeaxanthin results in increased macular pigment density,

plant power

Nutritional scientists are currently discovering that, in addition to vitamins and minerals, there are many other substances in foods that contribute to health. We have heard about plant hormones, especially isoflavones (see page 124), but watercress also contains substances that appear to protect against cancer. One naturally occurring chemical called isothiocyanate is thought partly to ameliorate the cancerous effects of some substances in cigarette smoke. Smokers who ate 3 very large portions of watercress 3 times a day showed less lung damage – however, do not assume that watercress can prevent lung cancer.

which improves the ability to filter off blue light and protect against free-radical damage. Lutein and zeaxanthin may also protect against cataracts, a progressive fogging of the lens of the eye making it difficult to see.

Other good sources of these carotenoids are red peppers, maize (corn), peas, celery and tomatoes.

rich in vitamins

Because we usually eat watercress raw, we benefit from its high level of nutrients. Many of these leach out during cooking, but are retained in recipes such as soup, where the cooking liquid is eaten.

Watercress is a very good source of folates (see page 13). It is also quite a good source of other B vitamins, such as thiamin (B1), riboflavin (B2), niacin (B3), B6 and pantothenic acid (B5). It is also a very good source of vitamin C and contains some vitamin E, both powerful antioxidants that work with the carotenes in the plant to protect against cancer and heart disease.

To round off the good news about this wonder plant, it is also a reasonable source of NSP (fibre) and is almost fat-free, containing just a trace of natural oils.

a mine of minerals

Watercress is also a rich source (for a vegetable) of calcium, potassium and iron. In addition, it provides sulphur, chloride, magnesium, copper and tiny amounts of zinc.

Magnesium is often overlooked, but it is needed for many enzyme functions vital for health, for example, the release of energy from food, enabling B vitamins to work; for growth and repair of body cells; and in the transmission of nerve impulses around the body.

Watercress is a great ingredient for drinks. Liquidize the rinsed leaves, then dilute the juice 4 parts to 1 with milder juices like citrus, apple or another vegetable such as celery.

natural antibiotics

Substances in the natural oils present in watercress (and mustard) have also been shown to be natural antibiotics. Unlike medical antibiotics, these do not harm the beneficial bacteria that live in our digestive system (see page 16) and boost immunity. However, eating watercress cannot take the place of specific antibiotics prescribed by your doctor.

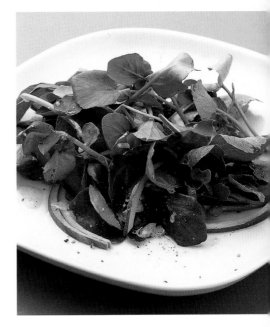

watercress soup

Silky smooth watercress soup makes a welcome lunch or light supper dish served hot in the winter and chilled in the summer.

preparation time **10 minutes**
cooking time **20 minutes**
serves **4**

1 onion, chopped
2 bunches of watercress, washed and trimmed
1 medium potato, diced, about 200 g (7 oz)
1 tablespoon sunflower oil
1 litre (1¾ pints) vegetable stock
125 ml (4 fl oz) natural yogurt (stirred) or
   single cream
sea salt and freshly ground black pepper
TO GARNISH
sprigs of watercress
freshly grated nutmeg

1 Sweat the onion, watercress and potato with the oil in a covered pan for about 7 minutes.
2 Add the stock and simmer for about 10 minutes, or until the vegetables are soft. Transfer to a food processor and liquidize to the desired consistency. Season to taste. Sieve for a finer consistency, if preferred, then reheat as necessary.
3 Either stir in the yogurt or cream and heat through (but do not allow to boil or the yogurt will curdle), or offer it separately. Garnish with sprigs of watercress and a grating of nutmeg. Serve with hot crusty bread.

salmon steaks with watercress mayonnaise

This is a very quick and easy dish to prepare and deceptively sophisticated when served! To further reduce the calorie content, use Greek-style yogurt instead of mayonnaise for the sauce.

preparation time **10 minutes**
cooking time **10–15 minutes**
serves **4**

4 salmon steaks, about 125–150 g (4–5 oz) each
4 teaspoons extra virgin olive oil
juice of 1 lemon
1 bunch of watercress
4 tablespoons reduced-fat mayonnaise
1 teaspoon Tabasco or other hot pepper sauce
   (optional)
sea salt and freshly ground black pepper

1 Place the salmon steaks on a layer of cooking foil in the grill pan and drizzle one teaspoon each of olive oil and lemon juice over each steak. Season with pepper and grill at a medium-high heat for about 5 minutes on each side.
2 While the salmon is cooking, put the watercress, mayonnaise and remaining lemon juice in a food processor and blend to a smooth sauce. Season to taste, adding the Tabasco, if using.
3 Keep the mayonnaise cold until ready to serve, then spoon over the hot fish and also, if liked, over any accompanying vegetables such as new potatoes and mange-tout or broccoli.

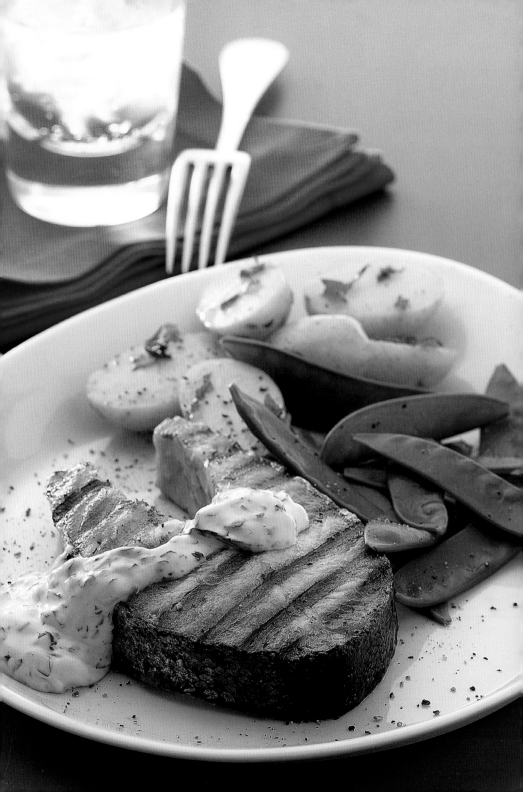

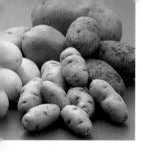

potatoes

Brought from Peru in the mid-1500s, potatoes have become the staple food of the West. The potato has certainly travelled well, both in culinary and nutritional terms.

POWER CONTENT

Vitamin B3
Vitamin C
NSP (fibre)
Calcium
Iron
Protein
GI 54 (crisps)
GI 62 (new)

PLUS POINTS

+ Immunity can be depressed by too much physical activity, but potatoes make a valuable contribution of immune-enhancing vitamin C to the sporting diet.

+ Excellent source of complex carbohydrates, with added fibre for slow-release energy if the skin is also eaten.

+ Sportspeople (or slimmers) will be interested to learn that new and cold potatoes provide a slower release of energy than those harvested from late summer onwards.

Potatoes are the epitome of power food. An excellent source of starchy, complex carbohydrate, they provide first-class energy to boost vitality. They give you the power to fight fatigue and boost immunity through their valuable contribution of vitamins and minerals and fibre. Niacin (vitamin B3) in potatoes also helps to maintain healthy nervous and digestive systems and is essential for normal growth and for healthy skin. Potatoes contain iron, calcium and protein.

We no longer mistakenly think spuds (and spaghetti and bread) are fattening, but know that starchy foods provide energy and are less likely to be laid down as body fat than fats and fatty foods. In fact, potatoes are fat-free and if kept that way can aid weight loss.

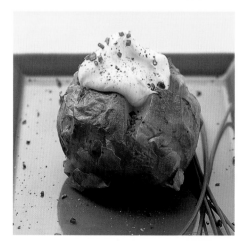

Reconstituted instant potatoes contain twice as much fibre as fresh mashed potatoes.

cooking to retain nutrients

How you prepare potatoes will influence how much of the vitamins and minerals are available to benefit your health. The way to retain nutrients is to cook potatoes in their skins and remove the skins after cooking, if necessary – remember that the skin on boiled and baked potatoes can be eaten. Avoid peeling, to conserve more vitamin C and fibre, and do not leave potatoes to soak in cold water before cooking, as the vitamins and minerals leach out. If you do peel them, do it as close to serving as possible and peel thinly, because most of the nutrients are just below the skin. Put the potatoes into the minimum amount of boiling water, as this shortens both the cooking and leaching time. Steam or microwave them for even greater savings.

potato calories   per 100 g (3½ oz)

crisps **533**	roast **157**	boiled **80**
chips average **250**	sauté **140**	instant mash **70**
oven chips **175**	baked **119**	
thick-cut chips **160**	mashed **105**	

surprising spuds

Despite their familiarity, potatoes do have some nutritional surprises for us. Their NSP (fibre) content makes them a valuable food and as we eat them in quantity the small amount of vitamin C can make an important contribution to the diet.

Amazingly, chips also have a lower GI factor (see page 8) than baked potatoes! This seems an argument for potatoes in their 'unhealthiest' form. In fact, the fat in the chips slows digestion and absorption from the stomach, lowering the GI factor – and too much fat is, of course, an important risk factor in heart disease. The same high levels of fat (plus salt and calories) can be found in crisps. So, while potatoes are a valuable staple food, it is important to eat the lower-fat versions of them on a daily basis.

Reheated potatoes and boiled cold potatoes (think potato salad) are also less easily digested and have the lowest GI!

New potatoes have a higher vitamin C level.

---

low-fat oven chips   serves 4 / 80 calories per portion

1 Boil 750 g (1½ lb) of potatoes cut into thick chips in about 1 litre (1¾ pints) of boiling stock and cook for 5 minutes, or until just tender.

2 Drain in a colander (reserving the stock for another batch of chips or to use in soup or sauces) and allow to cool slightly.

3 Put 2 tablespoons of vegetable oil in a large polythene food bag or box and carefully 'toss' the chips in the oil. (At this point you can freeze them for later use, once they are cold.)

4 Transfer the chips to a greased or nonstick baking sheet and bake in a preheated oven, 220°C (425°F), Gas Mark 7, for 10–15 minutes, turning once or twice,

until golden and crisp. If cooking from frozen, allow 15–20 minutes.

5 Sprinkle with paprika rather than salt.

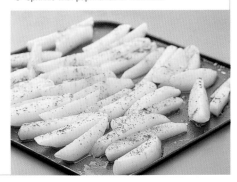

potato & prawn curry

Vary the degree of heat by using more or fewer chillies and adjust the ginger, ground coriander and cumin to suit your taste. Prawns are a treat, and this recipe makes a few go a long way.

preparation time **15 minutes**
cooking time **25 minutes**
serves **4**

1 tablespoon olive oil
1 onion, chopped
1 garlic clove, crushed
2 fresh green chillies, deseeded and chopped
1 green pepper, deseeded and chopped
5 cm (2 inches) fresh root ginger, peeled and grated
¼ teaspoon ground coriander
¼ teaspoon ground cumin
1 tablespoon white wine vinegar
500 g (1 lb) ripe tomatoes, skinned and chopped
500 g (1 lb) potatoes, scrubbed and cubed (no need to peel)
250 g (8 oz) cooked peeled prawns
15 g (½ oz) fresh coriander or parsley, chopped

1 Heat the oil in a large saucepan and sauté the onion, garlic, chillies, pepper and spices in the oil for 3 minutes. Do not allow to brown.
2 Stir in the vinegar, tomatoes and potatoes, cover with a lid, and continue to cook over a low to moderate heat, stirring occasionally, for a further 15 minutes.
3 Add the prawns and cook for 5 minutes more. Stir in the coriander or parsley and serve at once.

rösti florentine

preparation time **10 minutes**
cooking time **20 minutes**
serves **4**

1 kg (2 lb) potatoes, scrubbed
1 tablespoon lemon juice
50 g (2 oz) grated Parmesan cheese
6 tablespoons olive oil
250 g (8 oz) bag of spinach leaves
2 teaspoons butter
freshly grated nutmeg
4 free-range eggs
sea salt and freshly ground black pepper

1 Peel the potatoes (optional) and cut in half. Cook in boiling water for about 5 minutes, then drain under cold water to stop the cooking. Grate the potatoes, using a cheese grater or a rösti grater, which produces slightly larger grated potato pieces. Toss the lemon juice and Parmesan into the grated potato and season with salt and pepper. Separate the mixture into 4 equal-sized portions.
2 Heat 2 tablespoons of oil in a nonstick 22 cm (8½ inch) diameter frying pan. Put the individual röstis in the pan and flatten each one lightly, levelling the top. Cook for 5–7 minutes on one side. Remove the pan from the heat and and turn the röstis out on to a plate. Add another tablespoon of oil to the pan, return it to the heat, and when the oil is hot slip the röstis back into the pan to cook the other side. Both sides should be golden and crispy and the potato inside cooked.
3 While the röstis are cooking, rinse the spinach in cold water. Transfer it to a saucepan and cook over a moderate heat for 5 minutes – no need to add more water, but do use a well-fitting lid. Drain the spinach and return it to the saucepan, stirring in the butter and nutmeg to taste.
4 Poach the eggs by your usual preferred method and serve an individual rösti with spinach topped with a poached egg.

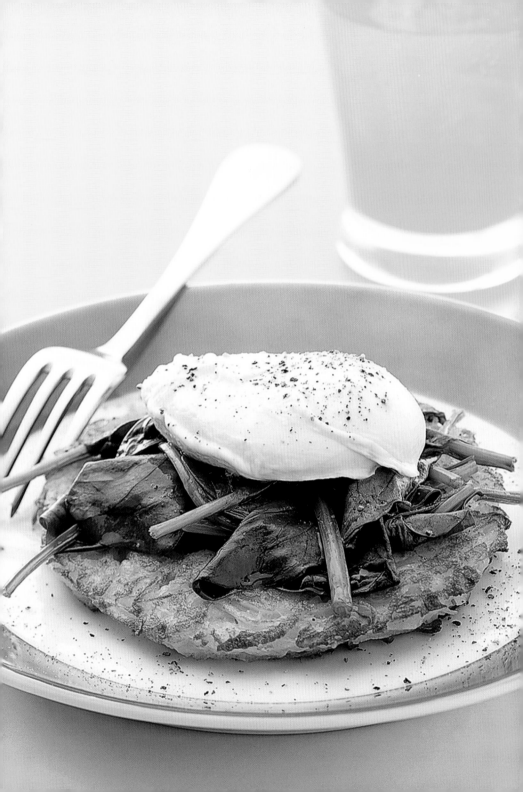

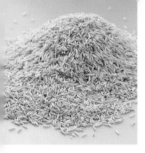

brown rice

Rice is the staple food of more than half the world's population. Most people eat white rice, but brown has many nutritional advantages and a unique flavour and texture. Rice is extremely versatile for cooking, and it is easier to make a wide range of low-fat healthy meals based around rice than around any other grain.

POWER CONTENT

Vitamin B
Vitamin B1
NSP (fibre)
Potassium
Magnesium
Zinc
Folates
GI 55–70

PLUS POINTS

+ **Wholegrain foods release their energy more steadily and cause fewer swings in blood sugar, a bonus for sportspeople.**

+ **Rice is a grain that is tolerated by virtually everyone, so if you have a gluten intolerance, or are sensitive to wheat, it makes an excellent alternative to wholemeal pasta (see page 68).**

Both white and brown rice first have the inedible husk removed from the grain after harvesting. Brown rice retains the bran layer and germ, which are removed when husked rice is polished to produce white rice.

Brown rice is available in both long- and short-grain varieties. Long-grain, as the name suggests, looks long and is thin with pointed ends. The grains should remain separate when cooked. Basmati is a prestigious variety of long-grain rice grown in the foothills of the Himalayas, prized for its aromatic flavour. American long-grain rice used to be called Carolina rice, from the area in which it is grown, but now it is grown in other areas. It is not as slim as basmati. Long- (and medium-) grain can be served with Asian dishes such as stir-fries and curries, or with fish, as the main starchy part of the meal. Also try jambalaya, pilau, biryani, pilaffs and rice salads.

nutrients in brown rice

Brown rice is a very good source of B vitamins, especially vitamin B1 (thiamin), which is needed to transmit messages between the brain and spinal cord. It is essential for enzymes that convert food into fuel for the body. Brown rice, unlike white, is also a good source of folates, vitamin E and NSP (fibre).

Eaten in combination with the other vegetable protein food groups (such as nuts and seeds or pulses), rice can also make a contribution to vegetarian protein. It is, however, lower in protein than wholemeal pasta.

Short-grain rice is also called round or pudding rice. It is plump and round in appearance, available in white and brown form, and can be used for risotto, paella and traditional rice pudding and other desserts. The authentic rice for paella is Valencia, a short-grain rice grown in the Valencia area of Spain, but sold only as white rice. Risotto rice, also only available as white rice, includes the Italian short-grain varieties Arborio and the more expensive Carnaroli, which absorb a lot of stock during cooking without becoming too soft and sticky. Short-grain rice is also used for rice pudding, rice moulds and for the Japanese dish sushi.

cooking rice

Rice absorbs a lot of water during cooking: 500 g (1 lb) absorbs about 600 ml (1 pint). It expands to twice its volume when cooked. Two heaped tablespoonfuls of boiled rice constitutes a serving (see the carbohydrate serving guidelines on page 18l), so allow one heaped tablespoon of uncooked rice per person. During cooking, starches are released that make the grains of rice stick together. This is desirable in some recipes, such as sushi, but can be avoided by rinsing the rice after cooking. Alternatively, rinse before you cook it: pour cold water over it and swirl around with your fingertips, then pour off the water; repeat until the water is clear. Do not rinse risotto or paella rice. Regardless of variety, all rice is cooked when the centre of the grain is tender.

Use the absorption method for long-grain or basmati, to give soft, fluffy grains. Measure both the rice and water accurately and use 1 part rice to 2 parts water. Simmer for 10–12 minutes, or until the water has been absorbed (about 30–35 minutes for brown rice). Remember that it is easy for the water to boil off too quickly and for the rice to burn on the base of the pan.

Easy-cook rice is partially cooked under pressure before milling. This has the nutritional advantage of driving some vitamins and minerals from the husk into the grain, but also slightly hardens the grain, making it slow to cook.

rice and GI

In general, rice has a high GI (glycaemic index) score, making it less beneficial for steady energy than pasta (which is probably why people complain that the white rice in a typical Chinese meal leaves them feeling hungry again relatively quickly). However, the GI score of rice depends on its amylose content. Amylose is a type of starch that is hard (like durum wheat, see page 8). Some rice contains more amylopectin, a softer starch than amylose, resulting in a higher GI score. In general, basmati rice has a higher amylose score than other rice, but published data for GI scores of white and brown rice vary. Brown rice has a slightly lower GI score than white rice. Parboiled or easy-cook white rice shares this marginal benefit with brown rice.

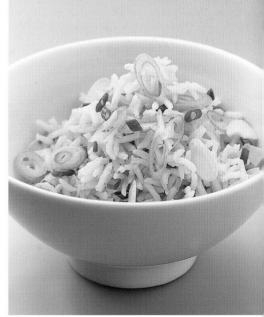

mushroom & celery risotto

Short-grain varieties of rice absorb a lot of stock during cooking without becoming soft and sticky. Brown rice is also firm enough not to become sticky, but it does not absorb as much liquid and takes longer to cook.

preparation time **15 minutes**
cooking time **30 minutes**
serves **4**

20 g (¾ oz) dried mushrooms (such as porcini, morels, ceps, champignons), sliced
2 tablespoons olive oil
1 garlic clove, crushed
1 large onion, chopped
2 celery sticks, chopped
100 g (3½ oz) fresh mushrooms, any kind
250 g (8 oz) brown rice
pinch of saffron
600 ml (1 pint) vegetable stock
freshly grated Parmesan cheese, to serve

1 Soak the dried mushrooms according to the packet instructions (usually a minimum of 15 minutes in boiling water).
2 Heat the oil in a large, heavy-based 20 cm (8 inch) saucepan and sauté the garlic, onion, celery and fresh mushrooms for about 5 minutes, or until softened.
3 Stir in the rice and cook for 5 minutes, stirring to prevent sticking. Add the saffron and the soaked mushrooms, including their soaking water (but be careful not to add any grit that has fallen to the bottom of the basin during soaking).
4 Stir in some of the hot stock and simmer for about 20 minutes. Stir occasionally, adding more stock until the rice has absorbed the stock and is cooked. Serve with grated Parmesan.

chicken biryani

This dish is started off on the hob and then transferred to the oven. It is a meal in itself, but it can be served with additional vegetables or a vegetable curry.

preparation time **20 minutes**
cooking time **40 minutes**
serves **4**

15 g (½ oz) butter
1 large onion, diced
2 garlic cloves, crushed
1 teaspoon grated fresh root ginger
2 fresh chillies, deseeded and diced
3 cloves
4 green cardamom pods
1 cinnamon stick
500 g (1 lb) boneless chicken, cut into thin strips
300 g (10 oz) brown basmati rice, washed
1 litre (1¾ pints) chicken stock
2 tablespoons chopped coriander leaves

1 Melt the butter in a casserole or dish with a lid that can be transferred from hob to oven. Add the onion, garlic, ginger and chillies and cook for 2–3 minutes while you pound the cloves and the seeds from the cardamom pods in a mortar.
2 Add the cloves, cardamom, cinnamon stick, chicken and rice to the pot and continue cooking for a further 5–7 minutes, turning the mixture occasionally.
3 Bring the stock to the boil and add. Cover with the lid and transfer to a preheated oven, 190°C (375°F), Gas Mark 6, for 30 minutes. When cooked, stir in the coriander leaves and serve.

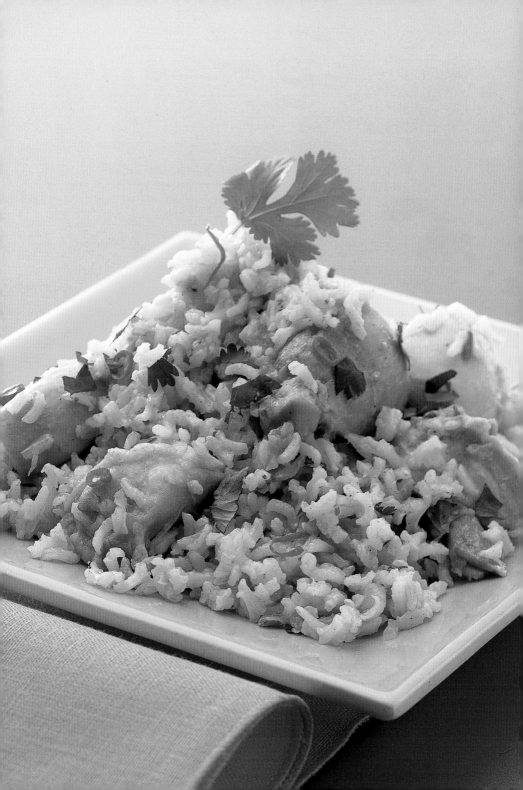

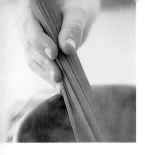

wholemeal pasta

Wholemeal pasta may have been seen as a food for 'cranks' in the past, but recent research into the speed at which food is digested confirms its value.

POWER CONTENT

B Vitamins
NSP (fibre)
Protein
GI approx 30–50

PLUS POINTS

+ Excellent for carbohydrate-loading, which is vital for endurance sports.

+ Wholegrain foods also release their energy more steadily and cause fewer swings in blood sugar.

+ Rich in B vitamins needed to cope with the stress of exercise – both physical and mental.

pasta for protein

Wholemeal pasta is also a good source of protein, though most people eat more than enough protein anyway. However, for vegetarians wholemeal pasta, eaten in combination either with nuts and seeds, or with beans or other pulses, will provide a vegetarian protein alternative to meat. Dairy food eaten with vegetable protein also enhances its usefulness to the body – so Parmesan cheese is a good accompaniment to pasta in more ways than one.

keep it healthy

Healthy cooking with pasta means retaining its low-fat profile. Serve it with a vegetable-based sauce, tossed in a spoonful of pesto or with a sprinkling of grated Parmesan cheese rather than with rich creamy or fatty meat sauces. It is just as delicious, and far lower in fat and calories.

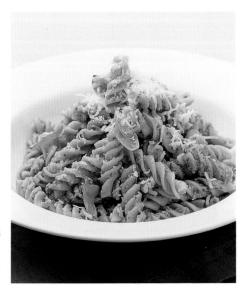

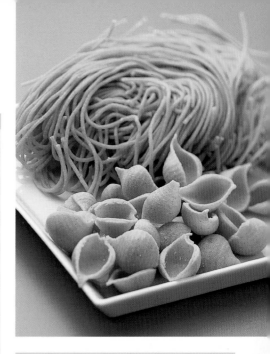

How much starchy food to eat

Most people need to eat 6 or more servings of starchy foods a day. This is so that these particular foods contribute around one-third of the total calories consumed.

A serving is measured as 3 heaped tablespoonfuls, or 45 g (2 oz), of boiled pasta. Details are given in the Introduction (page 18), but here is a more specific guidance:

Portions per day:

Age	Active females	Sedentary females
11–14	7–9	5–7
15–18	9–11	6–8
19–49	8–10	6–8
Women 50+	need 6–8 portions per day	

Portions per day:

Age	Active males	Sedentary males
11–14	9–11	7–9
15–18	10–14	9–10
19–49	10–11	8–10
Men 50–65	need 7–10 portions per day	
Men 65+	need 6–8 portions per day	

plain pasta

Some people find it very difficult to adjust to the taste of wholemeal pasta, and while it is definitely the best kind of pasta to eat, normal white pasta has its benefits too. Plain pasta still contains a sufficient amount of fibre and starch to be valuable, even though the flour used to make it has had the bran and wheatgerm removed.

wholegrain goodness

Wholegrain starchy foods – complex carbohydrates such as wholemeal pasta – still contain far more nutrients and beneficial substances such as NSP (fibre) and phytochemicals than refined (white) foods, irrespective of their relative GI values. For example, the undigested NSP from carbohydrate foods such as wholemeal pasta is ideal for encouraging a healthy digestive system, as beneficial bacteria thrive on it – too much sugar and too much meat encourage overgrowth of harmful types of bacteria.

cooking pasta

For fresh wholemeal pasta bring a large pan of water to the boil (how much depends on the quantity of pasta that you are cooking). Whether you add salt or not is a matter of personal preference, but a tablespoon of oil will help to keep the pasta shapes or strands separate. Add the pasta, bring the water back to the boil, then lower the heat to a simmer. Cook the pasta according to the instructions on the packet until it is al dente – tender but with some bite.

bacon penne

Penne, or quills, are a delightful shape for tossing in pasta sauce because the sauce seeps into the middle and clings all around the pasta, particularly if it is ridged.

preparation time **15 minutes**
cooking time **20 minutes**
serves **4**

2 celery sticks, diced
1 large onion, diced
2 garlic cloves, crushed
4 rashers of lean back bacon, diced
400 g (13 oz) can tomatoes
125 ml (4 fl oz) passata (sieved tomatoes)
300 ml (½ pint) vegetable stock
200 g (7 oz) wholemeal penne (pasta quills)
1 large carrot, grated
3 tablespoons chopped parsley
grated Parmesan cheese, to serve

1 Place the celery, onion, garlic and bacon in a pan, then cover and sweat for about 5 minutes without additional fat, stirring to prevent sticking.
2 Add the tomatoes and passata and cook for 10 minutes, breaking up the tomatoes as they cook.
3 Bring the stock to the boil and add with the pasta. Cook until the pasta is al dente.
4 Remove from the heat, stir in the carrot and parsley, and serve with grated Parmesan.

minestrone

The secret of a good-tasting minestrone is lots of fresh vegetables and not too much pasta. Elbow (bent) macaroni is often used, but wholemeal versions tend to be too big and chunky so break the thinnest wholemeal spaghetti you can find into small pieces.

preparation time **15 minutes**
cooking time **30 minutes**
serves **4**

2 tablespoons extra virgin olive oil
1 large onion, diced
2 garlic cloves, crushed
2 carrots, sliced
2 celery sticks, chopped
200 g (7 oz) French beans, halved
1 large courgette, chopped
500 g (1 lb) tomatoes, chopped
1.2 litres (2 pints) chicken or vegetable stock
300 g (10 oz) cooked or canned cannellini beans
75 g (3 oz) wholemeal pasta of your choice
4 tablespoons chopped parsley
1 rounded teaspoon celery salt
freshly ground black pepper
freshly grated Parmesan cheese, to serve

1 Heat the oil in a large heavy-based saucepan. Add the onion, garlic, carrots and celery and cook for 10 minutes, or until they begin to soften.
2 Add the French beans, courgettes and tomatoes. Stir well, then cover and cook for another 10 minutes.
3 Pour in the stock and bring to the boil. Cover the pan, reduce the heat and simmer for about 10 minutes.
4 Add the beans and the pasta and cook for another 10 minutes or until the pasta is cooked. Season, then stir in the parsley, celery salt and pepper. Serve with grated Parmesan.

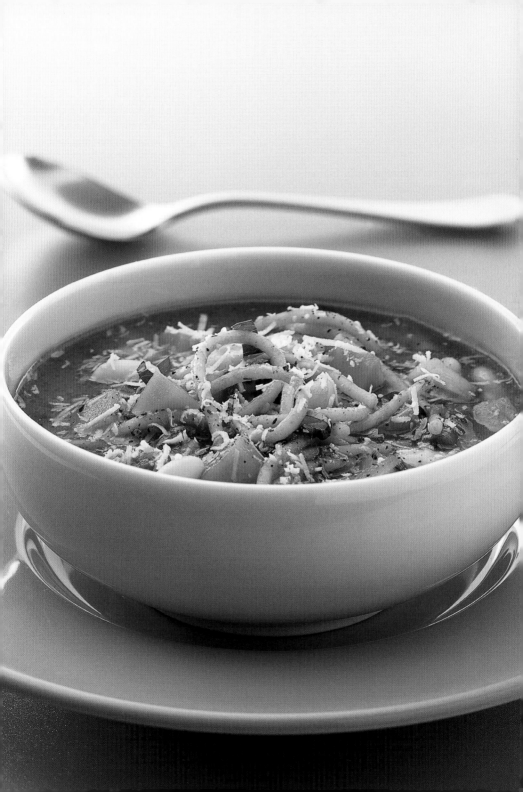

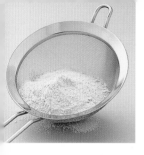

wholemeal flour

Wholemeal flour can be used in any recipe instead of white flour, but the results will be slightly different.

POWER CONTENT

Vitamin C
NSP (fibre)
Iron
Potassium
Sorbitol
Beta-carotene

PLUS POINTS

+ Wholemeal flour (unlike white flour) is an important source of B vitamins, needed for releasing energy from food.

+ A valuable provider of vitamin E, which is an antioxidant essential for a healthy heart.

+ Wholemeal flour also has a high fibre content which can act as a useful source of energy.

what makes wholemeal flour better for us?

The flavour of wholemeal flour is nuttier than white, and while this is prized in breads (see pages 76–77), its presence is greeted with less enthusiasm in cakes, biscuits, pastry and sauces. The difference between white, brown and wholemeal flours arises in the milling process. During milling, the wholewheat grain is crushed and ground to a flour. To make white flour, the germ (the seed or embryo) that contains most of the B vitamins and vitamin E is removed, along with the bran, which is the outer skin containing most of the fibre and the minerals iron and calcium. The wheatgerm and bran are left in wholemeal flour: it's 100 per cent of the grain. Brown flour has some of the bran and wheatgerm extracted and consists of between 85 and

flour power

Flour's strength refers to the quantity and quality of gluten-forming protein in the grain. In general, the more gluten there is, the stronger the flour. Stronger flours are recommended for bread, yeasted cakes and flaky pastry.

Medium strength (all-purpose) plain flour is suitable for most baking. Self-raising or 'extra fine' flour, which absorbs more fat and liquid than 'strong' bread-making and 'unbleached' flours, is good for cakes, biscuits and sauces. It produces a softer cake with a bigger crumb. Gluten is also present in barley, rye and oats, but not in the right quantity and quality to make them interchangeable with wheat flour in baking.

90 per cent of the original wheat grain. White flour has a 70–72 per cent extraction rate, and under British law white flour has to be fortified with calcium, iron and the B vitamins thiamin and niacin.

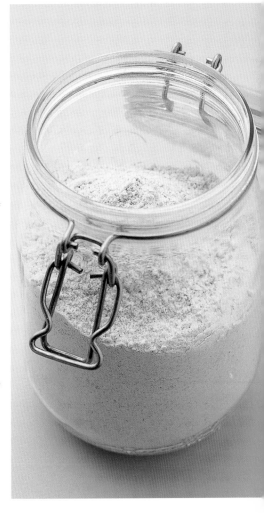

white flour

White flour lacks various vitamins and minerals essential for a healthy diet. It contains only 14 per cent of the vitamin E in wholemeal flour, 17 per cent of the magnesium and 17 per cent of the zinc.

cooking with wholemeal flour

Many people find that using a half-and-half mix of wholemeal and white is more acceptable, especially in cakes, particularly if wholemeal flour is unfamiliar. The main difference is in the density of finished baked goods. Wholemeal is heavier because it absorbs more water than white flour, and also because the bran and germ content prevent it rising as much. The differences are nothing to do with flour 'strength' (see box, left). Sifting adds air to baked goods and is particularly useful when working with wholemeal flour, but don't throw away the bran in the sieve, return most of it to the bowl. Adding baking powder or a mixture of cream of tartar and bicarbonate of soda in appropriate recipes gives a lighter finish. Substituted with 1 teaspoon of baking powder can be ¼ teaspoon of bicarbonate of soda and ½ teaspoon of cream of tartar.

plant hormones in whole grains

Whole grains contain lignans (see also page 101), a type of plant hormone that is present in cereals, legumes, vegetables and fruit. Grains contain up to 7 mg per 100 g (3½ oz) of lignans (fruit and vegetables contain up to 6 mg per 100 g). Linseed is exceptionally high, with around 60 mg per 100 g.

During digestion, lignans are broken down by friendly gut bacteria into structures that are interchangeable in the body for the female sex hormone oestrogen. They have both weak oestrogenic and anti-oestrogenic properties that protect against hormone-dependent cancers.

Fears about the phytate in bran in wholemeal flour interfering with absorption of minerals are probably unfounded as the body adjusts to any increase in wholegrain intake.

mix & match pizzas

preparation time **15 minutes, plus 2 hours proving for the dough**
cooking time **15 minutes**
makes **1 large pizza**

175 g (6 oz) flour, half-and-half unbleached plain
    white and plain wholemeal
2 teaspoons dried yeast
1 tablespoon extra virgin olive oil
100 ml (3½ fl oz) lukewarm water
125 g (4 oz) tomato-based pasta sauce
15 g (½ oz) basil leaves, torn
any other toppings of your choice, e.g. olives,
    anchovies, artichoke hearts (optional)
125 g (4 oz) mozzarella cheese, thinly sliced

1 Sift the flour into a mixing bowl, returning the bran
   from the sieve to the bowl.
2 Stir the yeast and oil into the water and keep stirring
   until the yeast has dissolved.
3 Make a well in the centre of the flour and stir in the
   yeast mixture using a fork. When combined, remove
   the dough from the bowl with floured hands and
   knead for 5 minutes. Return the dough to an oiled
   bowl or bag and leave in a draught-free place until
   doubled in size (up to 2 hours).
4 Return the dough to a floured surface and knock
   back (in other words, knead out the air). Knead again
   and roll out to the size of a dinner plate.
5 Place on an oiled pizza dish or baking sheet and
   spread over the tomato sauce. Sprinkle over the torn
   basil leaves and the toppings of your choice, then
   top with the mozzarella.
6 Place in a preheated oven, 220°C (425°F), Gas
   Mark 7, for about 15 minutes, or until the dough has
   risen and crisped and the cheese has melted.
7 Serve with a crisp green salad.

waffles with mixed berries

preparation time **15 minutes**
cooking time **15 minutes**
serves **4 (makes 8 waffles)**

75 g (3 oz) unsalted butter
2 free-range eggs
125 ml (4 fl oz) milk
125 g (4 oz) self-raising wholemeal flour
3 tablespoons icing sugar, sifted
grated rind and juice of ½ a lemon
450 g (14½ oz) pack of frozen mixed
    berries, defrosted
1 mint sprig, plus more to garnish
crème fraîche, to serve

1 Melt the butter, then allow to cool a little.
2 Separate the eggs. Add the yolks to the milk and
   whisk lightly. Add 1 tablespoonful of the melted
   butter to the milk and work in lightly with a fork.
3 Heat a waffle iron on the hob or preheat an electric
   one while you sift the flour into a bowl, returning the
   bran from the sieve to the bowl. Make a well in the
   flour and gradually beat in the milk and remaining
   butter. Whisk the egg whites until they are stiff
   enough to hold firm peaks, then fold into the batter
   together with 2 tablespoons of icing sugar and the
   lemon rind and juice.
4 Grease the waffle iron and pour in about one-eighth
   of the waffle batter. Close the lid and cook for 4–5
   minutes, turning the iron once or twice if using a
   hob model. When the waffle is golden brown and
   cooked, cover and keep warm while you cook the
   remaining waffles.
5 Put the fruit into a saucepan with the mint and heat
   gently until the juices run, stirring often to prevent the
   fruit sticking.
6 Put two waffles on each plate and top with some
   of the fruit. Shake over a little sifted icing sugar and
   add a mint sprig to decorate. Serve with crème
   fraîche, reduced-fat if preferred.

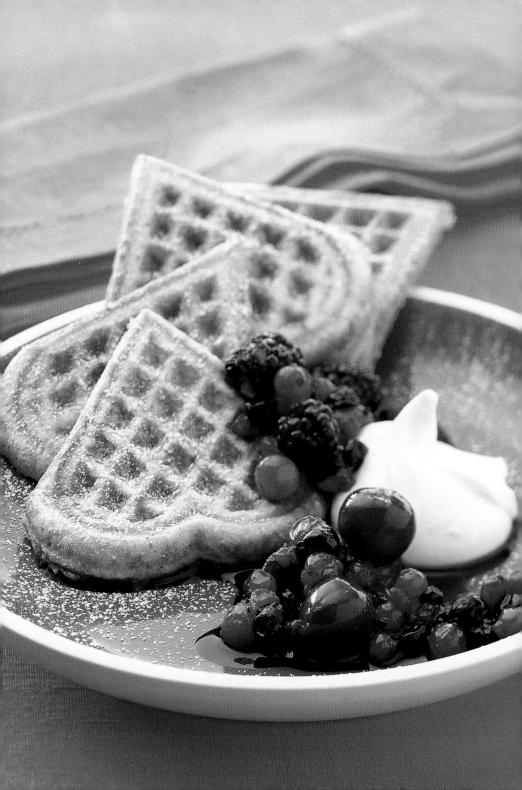

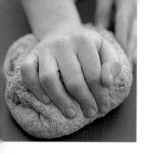

bread

'Give us this day our daily bread' is a familiar line to those who know the Lord's Prayer. 'May your rice bowl always be full' is as familiar an exchange among speakers of Mandarin Chinese, the language spoken by more people than any other. Both sayings recognize the importance of our daily staple foods.

POWER CONTENT

Vitamin B1, B3 and B6
Vitamin E
NSP (fibre)
Calcium
Iron
Zinc
Magnesium
Folates
GI 69 (wholemeal)

PLUS POINTS

+ White bread contains more calcium than wholemeal, essential for muscle contraction, part of all physical activity. The GI of white bread is 70–95.

+ Bread is a starchy food that releases energy more steadily than sugary foods, causing fewer swings in blood sugar.

+ Wholemeal (and other wholegrain) bread is an important source of B vitamins that release energy from food.

There are major nutritional differences between white and brown bread; wholemeal bread is superior in many respects. That said, all bread is good. Eating sufficient starchy foods, or using them to replace high-fat and high-sugar foods in the diet, is more significant than which bread you eat. It is important to enjoy food, and you can eat a range of breads (white and wholegrain) within a healthy diet – try to choose high-fibre kinds whenever you can. These are wholemeal, wholegrain, mixed grain, brown or 'high-fibre' varieties of bread.

nutritional value of wholemeal bread

Wholemeal bread is a good source of vitamin B1 (thiamin), which is needed to transmit messages

snack happy

Bread, regardless of its salt content, which varies widely, is a healthy snack, so eat sandwiches rather than a bag of salty crisps. A filled bread roll in a lunchbox is a far healthier choice than high-fat sausage rolls or fatty meat pies.

where white bread wins

White and brown bread contain more calcium than wholemeal as white flour is fortified with calcium (and iron, thiamin (B1) and niacin (B3)). It is vital for healthy bones and teeth, muscle contraction and the blood-clotting mechanism.

power source

Bread belongs to the starchy food group that should make up around one-third of your diet. Bread, like pasta, potatoes, rice and other cereals, is the best food source of energy. It also contains B vitamins to release that energy and support healthy nerves and digestion. As you will remember, 6 or more servings a day are recommended in a healthy diet (see page 18).

between the brain and spinal cord, and is essential in creating the enzymes that convert food into fuel for the body. Wholemeal bread also supplies niacin (B3), which is vital for releasing energy from food into the tissues and cells. It helps to maintain a healthy nervous and digestive system and is essential for normal growth and healthy skin. Vitamin B6 is important in protein metabolism. It promotes healthy skin and is absolutely vital for the maintenance of the nervous system. It is also needed for the formation of haemoglobin in red blood cells and of antibodies that help fight infection. Folates (see page 13) and vitamin E (for more see pages 88–89) are also found in wholemeal bread.

Wholemeal bread and other wholegrain breads provide more zinc than white and brown breads. Zinc is an important component of many enzymes, including superoxide dismutase (a powerful antioxidant enzyme that neutralizes potentially damaging free radicals). It is also required for growth, for immune-cell function and for healthy hair, skin and nails.

Unrefined cereals and wholemeal bread are an important source of magnesium, which works with calcium, and is needed for the formation in the body of many enzymes that facilitate the release of energy from food. It is also vital for the nervous system and muscle movement and for the formation of healthy bones and teeth.

The selenium content of wholemeal bread is good, but the amount varies depending on the soil where the grain was grown. Selenium is an important antioxidant.

We even obtain a significant amount of protein from bread, because we eat it so frequently and in combination with other vegetable food groups such as beans and pulses (beans on toast) and nuts and seeds (peanut butter sandwiches).

to be taken with a pinch of salt

Bread is sometimes described as a food that is high in salt. And, depending on the recipe, it can be. Breads such as soda bread and focaccia, with its visible salt crystals on the surface, are obvious contenders, but in most bread the salt content is hidden. Currently, food manufacturers, including bakers, are being urged to reduce the amount of salt added to staple foods such as bread. In many instances, bakeries have indeed reduced the amount of salt used – but they could do better! However, bread should not be avoided (unless on doctor's orders) as it provides other powerful and protective nutrients. Of course, if you make your own bread you can control the salt content.

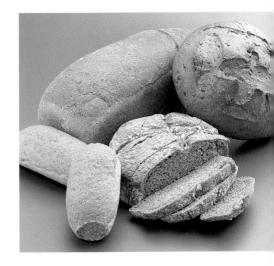

cinnamon & raisin bread & butter pudding

This is a delicious twist on the classic bread and butter pudding recipe. Using vanilla extract and brown sugar gives the dish a coffee-coloured appearance, but the flavour and aroma are fabulous.

preparation time **15 minutes**
cooking time **35–40 minutes**
serves **4**

4 slices of cinnamon and raisin bread
40 g (1½ oz) butter
2 free-range egg yolks
25 g (1 oz) brown sugar
½ teaspoon ground cinnamon
½ teaspoon vanilla extract
400 ml (14 fl oz) milk

1 Lightly butter a shallow ovenproof dish about 20 x 15 cm (8 x 6 inches) and a volume of just over 1 litre (1¾ pints).
2 Spread the bread with the butter. Cut the slices diagonally into halves and arrange in the dish, buttered side up.
3 Beat together the egg yolks, sugar, cinnamon, vanilla extract and milk. Pour over the bread.
4 Place the dish in a bain-marie (a roasting pan of hot water to come half-way up the sides of the dish) and bake in a preheated oven, 180°C (350°F), Gas Mark 5, for 35–40 minutes, or until the top is golden, the bread should look crispy and toasted and the custard should be set.

tomato, mozzarella & basil bruschetta

preparation time **15 minutes**
cooking time **4 minutes**
serves **4**

2 loaves of day-old ciabatta bread or pan toscano
6 ripe plum tomatoes, thinly sliced
1 garlic clove
2 tablespoons olive oil
a few sprigs of basil
125 g (4 oz) pack of mozzarella cheese,
    thinly sliced
sea salt and freshly ground black pepper

1 Cut the ciabatta into thick slices. Heat a cast-iron ridged griddle pan and put the bread on to 'toast', so that it gets almost burnt on the ridges of the pan. Do both sides. Allow to cool.
2 Skin the tomatoes: plunge them into boiling water for 1 minute, then remove and plunge into cold water. The skins should now peel off easily. Cut in half and remove the seeds and pulp. Dice the flesh.
3 Cut the garlic clove in half and rub the cut sides over the toasted bread. Sprinkle lightly with salt and spoon over the tomato, then drizzle with oil. Strew over some torn basil and then top with the mozzarella.
4 Place under a preheated hot grill and toast for about 4 minutes, or until the cheese has melted.
5 Drizzle over more olive oil, if liked, and garnish with more freshly torn basil leaves and freshly ground black pepper.

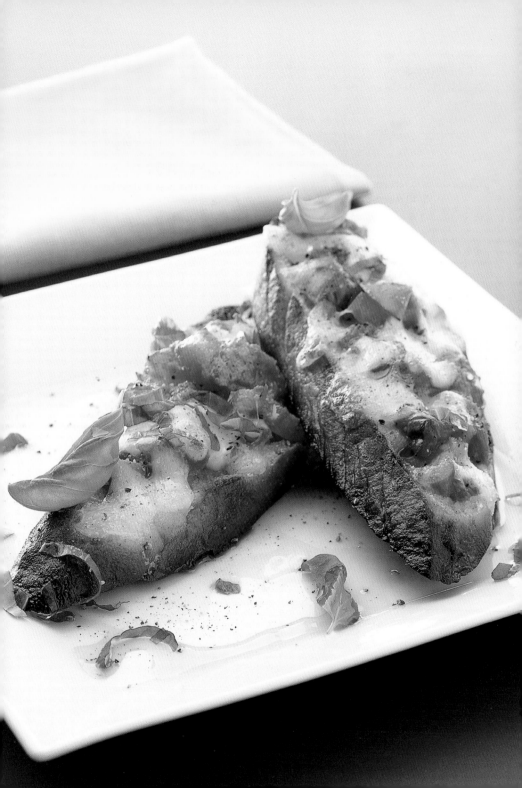

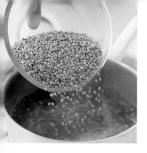

buckwheat

Buckwheat, with its sweet nutty flavour, is a traditional Russian staple that fits many modern dietary needs. It is quick to cook, tasty, versatile and rich in certain vitamins and minerals.

POWER CONTENT

Vitamin C
NSP (fibre)
Iron
Potassium
Calcium
Iron
Protein
Rutin
GI 54

PLUS POINTS

+ Ideal for a pre- or post-exercise light meal, such as a buckwheat salad or in place of couscous, as it is quick to cook.

+ A great source of energy for those who wish to avoid wheat: despite the name, it's not related to wheat and is gluten free.

+ As a good source of iron, buckwheat can help prevent lack of energy due to anaemia.

We think of buckwheat as a grain, but it is actually the seed of a plant that is related to rhubarb and dock. It is small, dark and triangular and takes about 15 minutes to cook. It can take the place of rice or other grains as a carbohydrate accompaniment to meat and fish, and can be used to stuff vegetables or make buckwheat equivalents of risottos and pilafs. Buckwheat probably originated in China and it has been a staple of Russian cookery for many generations now, where it was traditionally slow-cooked in an earthenware pot in the heat of a Russian stove.

getting a taste for it

A much nuttier flavour is achieved if the seed, or groat, as it is called, is dry-roasted in a frying pan over a

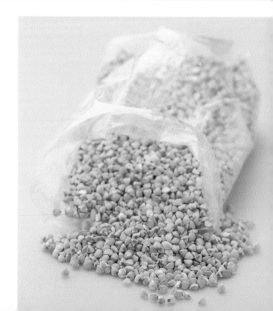

Buckwheat has a low GI score
(see page 8) when the whole
grains are cooked and served
as rice; when ground into flour,
the score is likely to be higher.

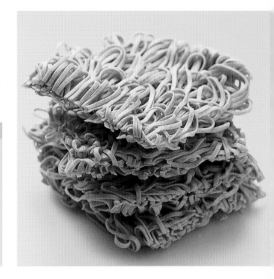

sprouting buckwheat

Occasionally, unhulled buckwheat groats can be
found in health food and other specialist stores.
These can be sprouted without first being
soaked. The hulls may fall away when the seeds
have grown large enough to eat; remove them if
not, because unlike most other sprouted seeds,
they are too tough to eat in salads or stir-fries.

moderate heat for about 10 minutes before being
steamed or boiled and served like rice. Alternatively the
roasted 'cereal' can be cooked into Kasha, a traditional
porridge-like Russian dish. Although traditionally eaten
as a main course accompaniment, you could try it for
a nutritious pre-training light meal or as breakfast
porridge: add chopped dried fruit, although it is already
quite sweet in flavour.

buckwheat flour

Hulled buckwheat groat is also ground into buckwheat
flour, which is made into pancakes. In Brittany, northern
France, buckwheat crêpes (pancakes) are popular.
They are usually large, thin and lacy and are made on
a big flat griddle. Their flavour is savoury. Buckwheat
flour is also made into a special type of Japanese
noodle called soba, available from health shops and
ethnic grocers.

In Russian cookery, buckwheat flour was traditionally
used to make blinis, small yeasted pancakes that are
cooked in a special buttered blini pan. Rather like a
wok, the blini pan is seasoned and then never washed,

just wiped out and cleaned with salt. The blinis are
traditionally dipped in melted butter or topped with
soured cream and black caviar – you could substitute
reduced-fat crème fraîche for a lower fat version of the
same recipe. They can be topped with pickled herring
or smoked salmon – a great way to enjoy oily fish.

pump up the iron

Buckwheat is rich in iron for a plant food (a little
more than spinach), and contains considerably
more calcium than rice. It is also a good source
of B vitamins and a very good source of rutin.
This is a type of bioflavonoid that strengthens
blood capillary walls and works with vitamin C.
Other foods that are good sources of rutin, such
as citrus fruits (see pages 36–37) and green
pepper, have higher vitamin C levels.

Two tablespoons of boiled buckwheat
constitute a serving if you are aiming to include
it in your 6–14 servings of starchy carbohydrate
foods per day (see page 18).

buckwheat noodle
& chicken chop suey

Buckwheat noodles have a pleasant texture that is more interesting than plain egg noodles. The flavour blends well with the oriental vegetables and chicken.

preparation time **15 minutes**
cooking time **20 minutes**
serves **4**

175 g (6 oz) buckwheat noodles
3 tablespoons vegetable oil
400 g (13 oz) boneless chicken, cut into thin strips
2 teaspoons cornflour
100 ml (3½ fl oz) soy sauce
¼ teaspoon ground ginger
1 tablespoon wine vinegar
juice of 1 orange
150 ml (¼ pint) water
200 g (7 oz) pak choi leaves, shredded
200 g (7 oz) bean sprouts
4 spring onions, sliced
250 g (8 oz) canned bamboo or water chestnuts, thinly sliced

1 Put the noodles on to boil or steam for 5 minutes or according to the packet instructions. Drain.
2 Heat 2 tablespoons of the oil in a wok or a large pan and fry the chicken for 5 minutes.
3 Mix together the cornflour, soy sauce, ginger, vinegar, orange juice, water and the rest of the oil to make a smooth sauce.
4 Add the vegetables and sauce to the pan and cook, stirring occasionally, for another 10 minutes.
5 Mix in the noodles, heat through and serve.

breton crêpes

Breton crêpes are thin and lacy and have a distinct flavour that is more savoury and nuttier than pancakes made with wheat flour. Even so, they are suitable for sweet or savoury toppings and fillings.

preparation time **15 minutes**
cooking time **1 minute each crêpe, or 15–20 minutes for the batch**
makes **about 15 small (12 cm/5 inch) pancakes**

2 free-range eggs
1 tablespoon vegetable oil
100 ml (3½ fl oz) cider or beer
125 g (4 oz) buckwheat flour
175 ml (6 fl oz) water
vegetable oil, for cooking

1 Lightly beat the eggs, oil and cider or beer.
2 Sift the flour into a large bowl, then add the liquid gradually, whisking all the time to form a smooth batter. Thin with the water and whisk again.
3 Leave the batter to stand for 10 minutes.
4 To make the crêpes, brush a 14 cm (5½ inch) omelette, crêpe or heavy-based frying pan with vegetable oil. Heat, but not to the point that the oil smokes. Pour in enough batter to coat the base of the pan and quickly tip the pan from side to side to cover the base before the mixture sets.
5 Cook on one side for about 30 seconds, then slip a palette knife or a thin spatula underneath and flip over to cook the other side for 30 seconds.
6 Remove the crêpes from the pan, cover and keep warm. Serve with ratatouille if liked.

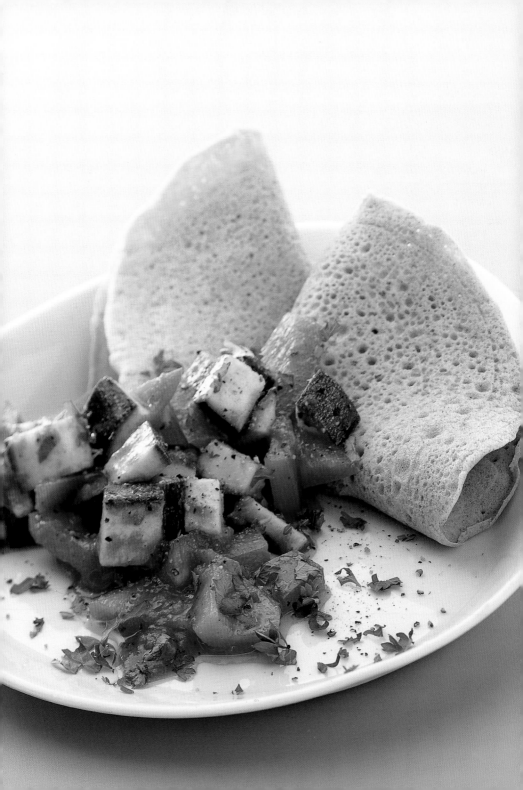

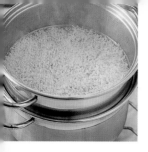

energy grains
burghul wheat & couscous

Burghul wheat is best known in its Middle Eastern incarnation tabbouleh. Though an 'old' ingredient, it is a brilliant modern convenience food, needing no cooking, just a quick soak.

POWER CONTENT	PLUS POINTS
Burghul B vitamins Calcium Iron GI 48	+ Burghul wheat is a good source of iron and B vitamins that helps prevent lack of energy due to anaemia. + Burghul wheat is not completely broken down during cooking, so it fuels endurance activities over time.
Couscous B vitamins NSP (fibre) Iron GI 65	+ Couscous provides a quick, but not long-lasting, fix of energy-rich carbohydrates.

burghul wheat

Burghul is a partially cooked cracked (kibbled) wheat. It is made by soaking the wholewheat grain, drying it in the sun then cracking it between rollers. Finally, it is hulled, steamed and roasted.

nutrition

Burghul has a lower protein content than buckwheat, to which it is comparable in a culinary sense, and it is due to this that it is considered to be another contributor to the starchy staple content of a healthy diet. Although it has only about a quarter of buckwheat's high calcium content, it is richer in iron, which is very useful for vegetarians and those who tend to have a low iron intake (most typically teenage and adult women). In addition, burghul is a good source of B vitamins.

cooking with burghul

In tabbouleh, burghul is mixed with chopped cucumber, mint and lemon juice. It can also be eaten like rice as an accompaniment, or added to soup. Burghul does not have to be cooked; it can simply be soaked in just-boiled water for about 10 minutes – be sure to put it in a large dish, as it swells and increases in volume while it absorbs the water. Use it in place of rice or mix it with vegetables.

In Middle Eastern cookery, burghul wheat is often used to make pilaf-style dishes. Vegetables such as

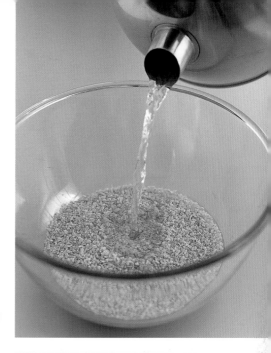

Because burghul wheat remains intact and is not completely broken down during cooking, it has the advantage of having a low GI score, providing energy in a steady stream that keeps you going for longer.

onions, garlic and peppers are sautéed in a pan, to which burghul is added, followed by stock. The mixture simmers over a low heat before being served, garnished with chopped mint.

Burghul is also easy to use in a wide variety of low-fat dishes – salads, fillings for stuffed vegetables and kibbeh. This gives it an advantage over pasta and potatoes, which can too easily turn into high-fat meals. Kibbeh are combinations of meat and bulgar, either mixed and formed into patties or with an outer shell of bulgar mixture and a filling of meat or pine nuts or walnuts. These are then baked.

COUSCOUS

Couscous is a cracked uncooked wheat, resembling semolina, which is popular in Moroccan, Tunisian and Algerian cooking. It is steamed over finely spiced broths and stews, usually of meat.

Couscous is made by taking pieces of semolina, the starchy central part of the wheat grain, and rolling them in fine flour. The coating is designed to keep the grains separate as they absorb the steam and swell over stews.

Vegetarian versions of the traditional stews are also popular today, and traditional meat stews sometimes contain added chickpeas and raisins. Harissa, a hot sauce made with cayenne or chilli pepper and pimento, is often served alongside couscous dishes.

Although couscous is traditionally bought uncooked, there are now precooked and partially cooked varieties

what's in a name?

A lot of unnecessary confusion can surround burghul wheat because it seems to have so many names. Other names for (and spellings of) burghul include: bulghur, bulgar, bulghul, pilgouri or pourgouri. Look for them in health food stores or Middle Eastern, Turkish or Greek shops.

available. These can be cooked in a matter of minutes or just rehydrated by adding boiling water. Precooked couscous contains fewer nutrients than traditional couscous. The trade-off for cutting down on cooking time is loss of most of the B vitamins, iron and fibre.

While couscous itself is not particularly nutritious, it is very low in fat and encourages consumption of vegetable stews. Like burghul, it can also be made into salads and pilaf-style dishes. It is traditionally cooked by steaming it in a couscousiére – with a meat tagine cooking underneath, all the goodness from the meat will rise and impregnate the couscous above. However, an alternative way to cook it, if this kitchen equipment is not available, is to line the top of an ordinary steamer with a piece of cheesecloth or muslin.

tabbouleh

A popular Lebanese dish that is both versatile and easy to make, tabbouleh can be served with meat and fish or as a salad in its own right.

preparation time **15 minutes**
cooking time **10 minutes**
serves **4**

250 g (8 oz) burghul wheat
½ –¾ cucumber peeled (optional),
    deseeded and chopped
4–6 spring onions, chopped
1 large handful of mint, chopped
1 large handful of parsley, chopped
2 tablespoons lemon juice
2 tablespoons olive oil
sea salt and freshly ground black pepper

1 Put the burghul wheat into a saucepan with enough boiling water to cover, then boil for 10 minutes. Drain if necessary and allow to cool.
2 Toss together the prepared vegetables and herbs, then mix with the burghul.
3 Whisk together the lemon juice, oil and seasoning and pour over the salad. Mix thoroughly.
4 Cover and refrigerate until needed, then bring to room temperature before serving.
5 Serve with pitta bread and hummus for a vegetarian meal, or use as an accompaniment to meat, fish and vegetarian savouries.

stuffed aubergines

preparation time **20 minutes**
cooking time **45 minutes**
serves **4**

2 aubergines
8 garlic cloves
2 lemons
6 tablespoons extra virgin olive oil
175 g (6 oz) pine nuts
250 ml (8 fl oz) water
150 g (5 oz) couscous
15 g (½ oz) butter
2 tablespoons chopped flat leaf parsley
2 tablespoons chopped coriander leaves
sea salt and freshly ground black pepper

1 Place the aubergines, whole garlic cloves and whole lemons in a shallow ovenproof dish with 1 tablespoon of the olive oil to prevent burning and sticking, and roast in a preheated oven, 180°C (350°F), Gas Mark 4, for 45 minutes.
2 Place the pine nuts on a separate baking sheet and lightly roast in the oven for 10 minutes.
3 Boil the water in a pan and add the couscous. Turn off the heat, stir in 1 tablespoon of the olive oil and the butter, and leave in the pan for 5 minutes.
4 When the aubergines, lemons and garlic are cool enough to handle, cut the aubergines in half lengthways and scoop out the soft pippy interior to leave a shell. Dice the flesh and put in a bowl. Scoop the centre from the lemons, removing the pips, and add to the bowl. Finally, remove the papery shell of the garlic cloves and add the flesh to the bowl.
5 Mash all the ingredients to a paste and mix in with the couscous and the chopped herbs. Season to taste. Pile the filling into the aubergine shells and sprinkle over the pine nuts. Drizzle over the remaining olive oil. Serve warm or at room temperature.

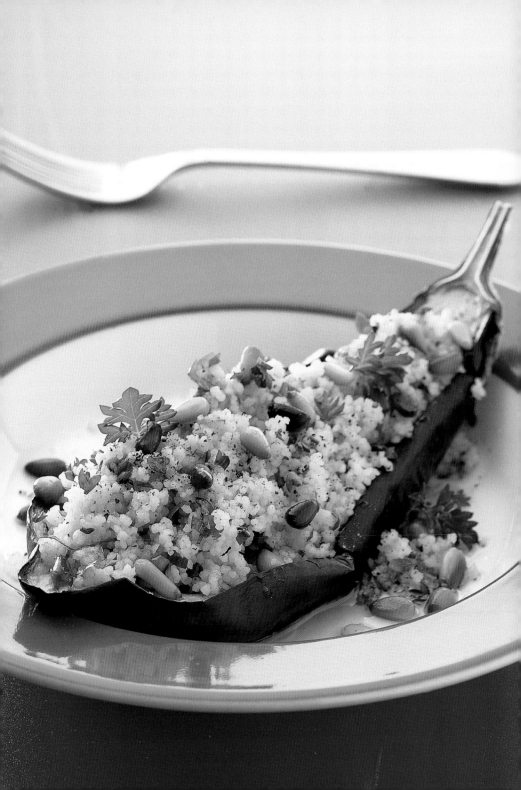

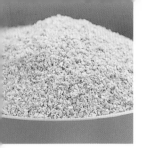

wheatgerm

Wheatgerm is made up of soft creamy flakes milled from the germ, which is the seed at the base of the wheat grain. As an embryonic plant, it is a nutritional powerhouse, rich in vitamins and minerals. It qualifies as a fast food, needing no cooking or preparation – just use it straight from the pack.

POWER CONTENT

B vitamins
Vitamin E
NSP (fibre)
Iron
Magnesium
Zinc
Folates

PLUS POINTS

+ A source of vitamin E, a powerful antioxidant for neutralizing the free radical effects of aerobic activity.

+ Wheatgerm also contains B vitamins for unlocking energy in food and making it available to fuel cells.

+ Iron, magnesium and zinc are also present in wheatgerm to assist muscle activity and prevent anaemia.

Wheatgerm is soft and appealing, with a deliciously appetizing cereal aroma. It is probably the most nutritious part of the wheat kernel: it contains most of the oils from the grain and is rich in protein, B vitamins and vitamin E.

In white flour the wheatgerm has been removed. Unless a bread is enriched with wheatgerm, there will be only a trace present.

nutritional benefits of wheatgerm

Vitamin E is hard to come by in useful amounts in most foods, making wheatgerm very valuable. One heaped tablespoonful of wheatgerm contains a little over 3 mg of vitamin E. Although there is no RNI for vitamin E (see opposite), government guidelines say that it is safe for women to eat 3 mg or more a day and men 4 mg or

more. Some dietitians translate these amounts as the nearest we have to a recommended adult's daily vitamin E requirement.

Wheatgerm is the reason that wholemeal flour (see page 72) and wholemeal bread (see pages 76–77) are good sources of vitamin B 1 (thiamin) and vitamin B2 (riboflavin). In addition, wheatgerm supplies vitamin B3 (niacin), vitamin B6, folic acid and the minerals iron, magnesium and zinc. Even though wheatgerm derives from the wholewheat grain, it is not in itself as good a source of NSP (fibre) as wholemeal flour or bread, although some fibre from the bran layer of the grain does remain attached to wheatgerm. Wheatgerm contains 2–2.5 g of NSP per 100 g (3½ oz). This is the same amount that is to be found in white bread, compared with 5 g found in brown bread and 8.5 g in wholemeal bread.

how much vitamin E do you need?

This is a difficult question. In the UK there is no official recommendation for the amount adults need, because it is said that requirements differ depending on fat intake. This means that the higher your polyunsaturate intake, the higher the need for vitamin E. However, the EU has an RDA (recommended daily amount) of 10 mg per day for adults. This coincides with the US and Canada, but is lower than the Australian figure of 10–15 mg. Bear in mind that these figures are for disease prevention, not optimum health. Leading medical experts on antioxidants suggest we need a much higher intake, 60–100 mg per day, for antioxidant protection. This amount is very difficult to achieve through diet. Analyses of the vitamin E content of wheatgerm vary, and you would need to eat 50–100 g (2–3½ oz) to meet the lowest recommendations of 10 mg per day.

the many ways with wheatgerm

Wheatgerm can be added to baked goods – some breads enriched with added wheatgerm have a characteristic soft, springy centre (the most famous being Hovis). It can be used in biscuits and cakes and other bakes, or sprinkled over cereals and yogurt or other desserts as a topping. Less conventional use is to add it to salads and soups. When used in home-made meat loaf and burgers, or vegetarian equivalents made from lentil and grain mixtures, it acts as a binder and extends the recipes without being intrusive in texture or flavour. It can also be mixed with herbs and spices for use as a coating, where breadcrumbs might otherwise be used, on fish or fishcakes, chicken or rissoles. It also makes delicious scones, as the recipes on the following page demonstrate.

protecting cells

Vitamin E is an antioxidant vitamin that helps to neutralize damaging free radicals in the body. It is particularly important for the protection of cell membranes, where it prevents the fats being oxidized and producing free radicals. It also helps maintain healthy skin, heart and circulation, nerves, muscles and red blood cells.

Vitamin E is used in many body processes to protect against oxidative damage and has therefore been linked to reducing the risk of many diseases, such as heart disease, stroke, cataracts and some cancers.

natural vitamin E

The benefit of the vitamin E in wheatgerm is that it is natural. Trials of vitamin pills have shown that the natural form of vitamin E, written on supplement bottles as d-alpha-tocopherol, is more beneficial than the synthetic version, dl-alpha-tocopherol.

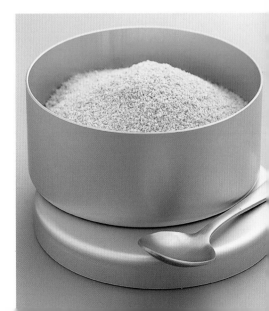

savoury wheatgerm scones

Savoury scones are very versatile. They make
excellent snacks, or can be served warm for
breakfast or as a supper dish.

preparation time **15 minutes**
cooking time **12–15 minutes**
makes **6–10 (depending on size)**

200 g (7 oz) self-raising white organic flour
125 g (4 oz) wheatgerm
pinch of salt
½ teaspoon bicarbonate of soda
½ teaspoon cream of tartar
15 g (½ oz) coriander or flat leaf parsley,
    finely chopped
40 g (1½ oz) butter
75 g (3 oz) grated Cheddar cheese
150 ml (¼ pint) soured milk
additional milk or single cream, for glazing

1 Lightly oil a baking sheet.
2 Mix the flour, wheatgerm, salt, bicarbonate of soda,
   cream of tartar and coriander or parsley.
3 Rub in the butter until the mixture resembles
   breadcrumbs in consistency.
4 Stir in the cheese, then mix in the soured milk using
   a fork to make a soft dough.
5 Turn out on to a gently floured board and knead
   very lightly to make a smooth dough. Pat down
   to a 2.5 cm (1 inch) thickness and cut out either
   6 large 7 cm (3 inch) or about 10 small 5 cm
   (2 inch) scones.
6 Place on the prepared baking sheet and brush with
   milk. Bake in a preheated oven, 220°C (425° F),
   Gas Mark 7, for 12–15 minutes, depending on the
   size of the scones. They are baked when they sound
   hollow if tapped on the base or when an inserted
   skewer comes out clean.

raisin & wheatgerm scones

Adding wheatgerm to scones gives them a very
pleasant soft texture and improves the depth
of flavour.

preparation time **15 minutes**
cooking time **12–15 minutes**
makes **6–10 (depending on size)**

125 g (4 oz) plain wholemeal flour
40 g (1½ oz) plain white flour
125 g (4 oz) wheatgerm
½ teaspoon bicarbonate of soda
½ teaspoon cream of tartar
40 g (1½ oz) butter
25 g (1 oz) golden caster sugar
75 g (3 oz) raisins
150 ml (¼ pint) soured milk
additional milk or single cream, for glazing

1 Lightly oil a baking sheet.
2 Mix the flours, wheatgerm, bicarbonate of soda and
   cream of tartar in a mixing bowl.
3 Rub in the butter until the mixture resembles
   breadcrumbs in consistency.
4 Stir in the sugar and raisins. Mix in the soured milk,
   using a fork, to make a soft dough.
5 Turn out on to a lightly floured board and knead
   very lightly to make a smooth dough. Pat down
   to a 2.5 cm (1 inch) thickness and cut out either
   6 large 7 cm (3 inch) or about 10 small 5 cm
   (2 inch) scones.
6 Place the scones on the prepared baking sheet
   and brush with milk or cream. Bake in a preheated
   oven, 220°C (425° F), Gas Mark 7, for 12–15
   minutes, depending on the size of the scones. They
   are baked when they sound hollow if tapped on the
   base or when an inserted skewer comes out clean.

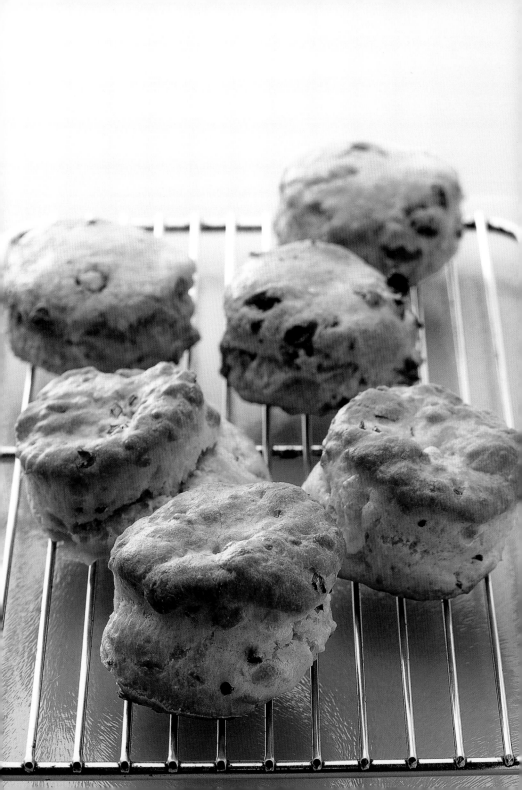

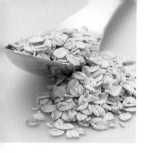

oats

Oats have been the power food behind the Scots for generations. But it is only recently that they have risen to nutritional fame with the discovery of 'soluble fibre'. Since then, oat products have been permitted to make claims that they can help reduce cholesterol, but that only works as part of a low-fat balanced diet.

POWER CONTENT

Vitamin B3
NSP (fibre)
Calcium
Iron
Lignans
Gluten-free
Unsaturated oils
GI 42 (porridge)

PLUS POINTS

+ **Super source of slow-release energy for endurance sports and physical activity in general.**

+ **Helps lower blood cholesterol levels and controls blood pressure – useful aids to heart health and physical fitness.**

+ **Higher in calories (due to natural oils) than many cereals, a bonus for endurance athletes.**

For oats to have an effect on blood cholesterol levels, they must be eaten on a regular basis as part of a well-balanced diet. The minimum to eat and still see an effect is around 40–50 g (1½ –2 oz) a day. That's the amount of oats found in a medium bowl of porridge or a large flapjack. Most studies have found 150 g (5 oz) a day to be a more effective amount to eat.

Oats reduce both total blood cholesterol and levels of harmful low-density lipoprotein (LDL) without reducing levels of beneficial high-density lipoprotein (HDL) levels. It is important to keep HDL levels high to protect against heart disease. Eating more oats and oat products (along with enough fruit and vegetables) displaces potentially salty foods and increases fibre, which can lower blood pressure.

Lignans (see page 101), which are similar to the beneficial isoflavones found in phytoestrogens, are also to be found in oat bran and oatmeal.

fashion for fibre

When the fashion for high-fibre foods arose in the early 1980s all attention focused on wheat bran. Subsequently it was realized that the bran is mainly insoluble but that fibre in oats and beans (and other legumes) is mainly soluble. A healthy diet requires a mix of both types of fibre. You need the bran fibre for regular bowel movements. It promotes growth of bacteria that make a soft and bulky stool. Efficient digestion and evacuation prevent diverticular disease, haemorrhoids and varicose veins.

The gummy fibre in oats and beans acts in a different way. It lowers cholesterol levels and regulates

> If you want to boost your NSP (fibre) intake with a product that has a low GI (see page 8), try partial substitution of oat bran for flour when baking.

the sugar levels in blood, thus reducing the chances of developing diabetes. Gummy fibres also help lower blood pressure. Soluble fibre reduces cholesterol in two ways. First it increases the loss of bile acids. These are made from cholesterol in the liver and are needed for the digestion of fat. Gummy fibre increases the excretion of bile acids in faeces, thereby lowering blood cholesterol. Bacteria in the colon also ferment soluble fibre to produce acids that travel to the liver, where they turn off cholesterol production. This is a significant advantage since it is cholesterol that clogs arteries, causing them to narrow and harden, which can contribute to a heart attack.

perfect porridge

Porridge, made either from oatmeal or rolled oats, is a hot and filling meal (like breakfast cereal) at any time of the day or night. Make it with milk or with water, depending on personal tastes. Traditionally, salt is added, but dried fruit, such as raisins or chopped dates, can be stirred in during or after cooking to sweeten. Alternatively, sweeten the porridge to taste at the table with sugar (the least 'healthy' option), maple syrup,

oats so good

The process of milling oats is not very intensive, so they retain a high percentage of their nutrients. After the outer husk is removed, the inner groat is ground and cut into several pieces known as pinhead meal, which is ground further to make fine or medium oatmeal. For porridge oats, the groats are flattened between heavy rollers.

For a plant food, oats are a good source of the minerals calcium and iron. They are a good source of the vitamin niacin (B3). They contain more protein than other common cereals and are higher in oils and calories.

the making of muesli

In the early 1900s, Dr Max Bircher-Benner, the Swiss nutritional therapy pioneer, invented muesli, which came to epitomize healthy eating. Originally made from coarsely milled wholewheat grains in milk, it was sweetened with honey and fruit: grated apple or strawberries or bilberries.

Birchermuesli was later modified to include oatmeal. It was soaked overnight in milk or apple juice to soften and swell the grains and make them more digestible. Muesli now invariably contains oats.

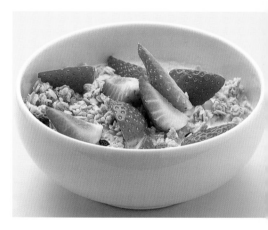

molasses or black treacle. Porridge is a brilliant healthy fast food, which can be made quickly in a jug in a microwave oven.

Traditional porridge has a low GI (see page 8). but 'one-minute' oats and similar products have an intermediate GI because the groats have been milled to a far finer grade, then pre-cooked and rolled very thinly, increasing the rate at which they can be digested. Porridge is suitable for people who cannot tolerate gluten and therefore cannot eat standard breakfast cereals.

treacle oat crunchies

These biscuits are very simple to make and have a pleasant texture. The treacly flavour is reminiscent of toffee and liquorice. Store in an airtight tin and serve with ice cream or fruit or in packed meals.

preparation time **15 minutes**
cooking time **about 12 minutes**
makes **16**

125 g (4 oz) butter or margarine
100 g (3½ oz) golden caster sugar
1 teaspoon vanilla essence
2 tablespoons black treacle
125 g (4 oz) self-raising organic plain white flour
75 g (3 oz) organic plain wholemeal flour
125 g (4 oz) porridge oats

1 Grease 3 baking sheets.
2 Melt the butter or margarine and sugar in a saucepan or microwave jug. Stir in the vanilla essence and treacle.
3 Mix the flours and oats in a bowl and stir in the melted ingredients.
4 Form into 16 balls, put on to the baking sheets and flatten slightly with the back of a fork. Bake in a preheated oven, 180°C (350°F), Gas Mark 4, for 12 minutes, or until slightly risen and well-coloured.

crunchy oat fruit crumble

Crumble toppings for fruit puddings can be disappointingly soft and soggy, but this one is crisp and crunchy and more like a granola topping.

preparation time **15 minutes**
cooking time **30 minutes**
serves **4**

500 g (1 lb) prepared rhubarb, apples, plums or
    other fruit of your choice
50 g (2 oz) sugar (optional)
3 tablespoons water
75 g (3 oz) butter or margarine
125 g (4 oz) demerara sugar
1 tablespoon golden syrup
250 g (8 oz) porridge oats
50 g (2 oz) plain wholemeal flour

1 Wash and slice the rhubarb or peel, core and slice the apples and place in a saucepan with the sugar (optional) and the water, which should be enough to just cover the base of the pan to prevent the fruit sticking and burning. Cover and heat gently for 10 minutes to partially soften the fruit. Drain off the excess cooking juice and transfer the fruit and some juice to a 1.5 litre (2½ pint) ovenproof dish.
2 Melt the butter with the sugar and syrup, then remove from the heat and stir in the oats and flour. Spoon over the fruit. Do not press down, but leave the crumbed mixture loosely covering the fruit.
3 Place in a preheated oven, 180°C (350°F), Gas Mark 4, and bake for 20 minutes, or until golden brown. Serve the crumble with custard, if liked, or a thick natural yogurt.

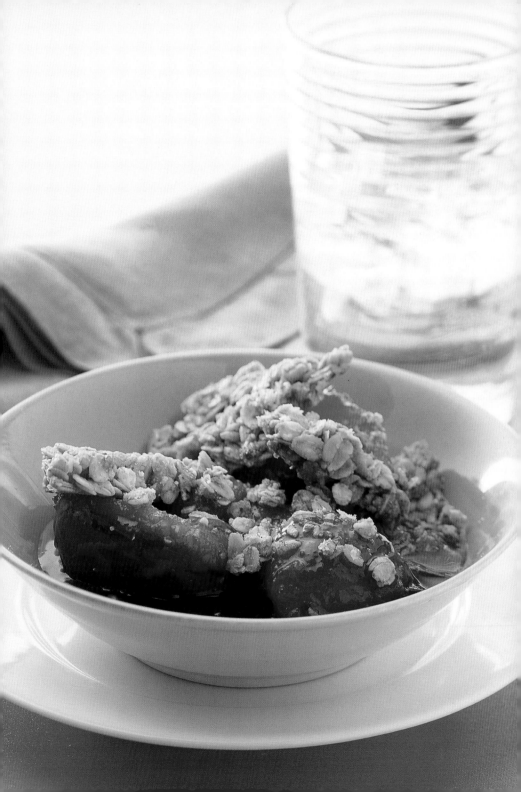

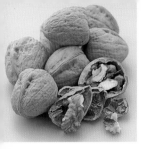

nuts

Treat nuts right and they will reward you. Elevate them from a party nibble, or an accompaniment to aperitifs, to main meal status. That way you benefit from them as a nutrient-dense concentrated food source and not as a 'fattening' snack food.

POWER CONTENT

Vitamin E
NSP (fibre)
Magnesium
Potassium
Amino acids
Omega-3 fatty acids
Unsaturated fats
GI 14 (peanuts)

PLUS POINTS

+ One of the most concentrated sources of high-fibre food energy for sportspeople.

+ Nuts contain oils (which provide energy in addition to some carbohydrate content), in the form of unsaturated fats.

+ The high vitamin E and mineral content of nuts protects against antioxidant damage and other sporting stresses.

Nuts have an enormous amount to offer. They may be high in calories, but they are also packed with nutrients. The fat they contain is unsaturated and of the type that protects against heart disease. Nuts are also a good source of NSP (fibre). The sole exception is the coconut, including products like creamed coconut.

Salted nuts are not good news for people with high blood pressure, and the high calorie content may be problematic for those who need to lose weight. But if (unsalted) nuts are treated as a main source of calories and not eaten as a high-fat snack additional to normal calorie needs, they become 'superfoods'.

healthy heart

Research has shown that people who eat nuts frequently have a far lower risk of heart disease than those who do not eat nuts; intermediate nut consumers have an intermediate risk.

This could be due to a number of effects. The unsaturated fats in nuts could be helping to lower blood cholesterol levels, and/or their omega-3 fats may be preventing blood-clotting and harmful disruptions to heart rhythms. Nuts are a rich source of arginine, an amino acid that stimulates production of nitric oxide, which relaxes the cells that line arteries and also helps make blood less likely to be sticky and clot. Nuts also contain a lot of magnesium, potassium, NSP (fibre) and vitamin E, the latter a component of many enzymes that give antioxidant protection to body cells. In addition, the protective antioxidant minerals selenium, copper and folic acid are all evident in nuts.

getting the balance right

But it's not just about eating more of one type of polyunsaturate, the omega-3 type contained in nuts and oily fish (see pages 116–117). The balance between omega-3 and omega-6 fatty acids is important. Both families of fatty acids compete for the same enzymes to make them and because we eat a lot of omega-6 fats, the ratio in our diet is skewed towards omega-6. For better health, we need to shift from the current ratio of 7:1 to 6:1. Experts advise that the best way to correct the balance is to eat more nuts and oily fish.

Thirty years ago we had a healthier ratio. Our current greater intake of omega-6 over omega-3 is due to eating less oily fish and fewer nuts. There are also other factors: increased use of polyunsaturated oils and spreads; manufacturers are putting more vegetable oils into processed foods, and livestock from intensively farmed meat does not contain as much omega-3 as meat, poultry and eggs from organic or free-range grass-fed livestock. To obtain 4–5 g of omega-3 fatty acid you need to eat a 169 g portion of mackerel; 200 g sardines; 2 x 150 g salmon or trout; 4 x 90 g beef and 3 x 20 g walnuts.

omega-3 fatty acids for vegetarians

The richest sources of omega-3 fatty acids are oil-rich fish, but don't worry if you are a vegetarian or can't eat fish. If your diet does not contain too much saturated fat, the omega-6 fatty acids in green leafy vegetables, some nuts, some vegetable oils and some margarine / spreads can be turned into a similar fatty acid.

Eat more vegetables (particularly dark green ones) and walnuts and use rape seed or soybean oils for cooking and in salad dressings, because these all have a high alpha-linolenic acid content. Other foods that have a relatively high omega-3 to omega-6 ratio include linseed (see page 100) and linseed oil. Linseeds can be added to cereals and baked foods.

People who eat nuts frequently have a far lower risk of heart disease than those who do not eat nuts.

the 'walnut diet'

A 'walnut diet' trial in the US, published in The New England Journal of Medicine in 1993, saw 18 men aged 21–43 fed 84 g (about 3 oz) of unsalted and unroasted walnuts each day as a substitute for other high-fat foods in a typical American diet. The result was lower cholesterol levels, with a major reduction in LDL 'bad' cholesterol and only a minor decrease in HDL good cholesterol. As little as 28 g (about 1 oz) of walnuts per day has been shown to have a beneficial effect within one month, and a long-term 13-year study of vegetarians has shown a 23 per cent lower than average death rate among those who eat nuts regularly.

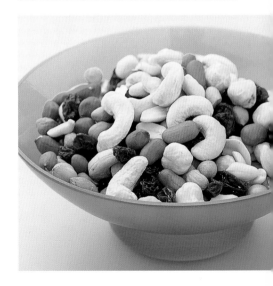

waldorf crostini

preparation time **15 minutes**
cooking time **15 minutes**
serves **4 as a snack or appetizer**

1 crisp apple, cored but not peeled
1 teaspoon lemon juice
2 celery sticks
50 g (2 oz) walnuts, coarsely chopped
½ Iceberg or similar crisp lettuce, shredded
150 g (5 oz) thick Greek-style yogurt
sea salt and freshly ground black pepper
FOR THE CROSTINI
2 tablespoons olive oil
4 thick slices of walnut bread
150 g (5 oz) goat's cheese
finely chopped walnuts, to garnish (optional)

1 Brush the olive oil on to the walnut bread and put
   them on a baking sheet in a preheated oven, 200°C
   (400°F), Gas Mark 6, for 10 minutes to crisp.
   Remove from the oven.

2 Cut the goat's cheese into 12 slices to fit on top of
   the crisped crostini and either return to the oven for
   4–5 minutes or melt the cheese by placing the
   crostini under a moderately hot grill.

3 While the crostini are cooking, make the salad. Dice
   the apple and mix with lemon juice in a bowl large
   enough to take all the ingredients. Add the celery,
   walnuts and lettuce. Season, then fold in the yogurt.

4 Place a generous mound of salad on each plate,
   and arrange one of the crostini beside it. Sprinkle
   the crostini with a small amount of extra chopped
   walnuts, if liked.

chicken skewers
with satay sauce

preparation time **20 minutes plus marinating**
cooking time **15 minutes**
serves **4**

4 boneless, skinless chicken breasts, cut into
   bite-size pieces
FOR THE CHICKEN MARINADE
150 g (5 oz) Greek-style natural yogurt
2 tablespoons finely chopped coriander leaves
1 teaspoon each ground coriander and cumin
black pepper
FOR THE SATAY SAUCE
1 stem of lemon grass, chopped
1 shallot, chopped
1 cm (½ inch) fresh root ginger, grated
2 fresh chillies, seeded and chopped
1 teaspoon chilli powder
2 tablespoons vegetable oil
3 tablespoons crunchy peanut butter
175 ml (6 fl oz) coconut milk
1 tablespoon dark brown sugar
juice of 1 lime

1 Mix together the marinade ingredients. Pour over the
   chicken, cover, and refrigerate for at least 2 hours.

2 Blend or process the lemon grass, shallot, ginger,
   chillies, chilli powder and vegetable oil to a paste.

3 Thread the chicken pieces on to skewers and grill
   over a high heat for about 15 minutes, turning often.

4 Brush the bottom of a heavy pan with the oil, then
   fry the spice paste for about 3 minutes over a
   medium heat, stirring. Add the peanut butter and
   blend well.

5 Reduce the heat and stir in the coconut milk, sugar
   and lime juice to make a thick sauce. Add boiling
   water if you want a thinner sauce.

6 Serve the chicken and satay sauce with rice and
   salads of mango and banana or chunky cucumber
   mixed with spring onions, coriander and wine
   vinegar.

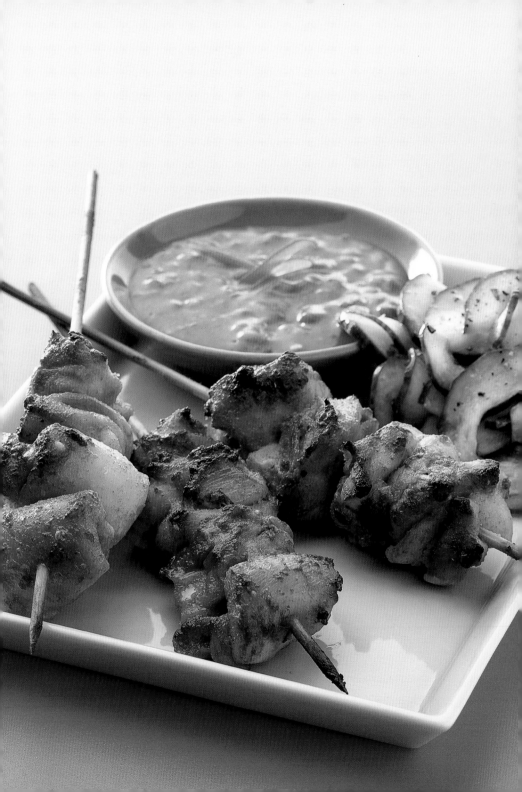

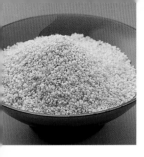

seeds

Seeds are a powerhouse of nutrients, as they contain all the goodness needed to sustain life while the next generation of the plant begins its growth. Although they contain fats, these are beneficial unsaturated oils.

POWER CONTENT

Vitamin C
Vitamin E
Amino acids
Iron
Calcium
Zinc
Lignans
Omega-3 fatty acids
Unsaturated oils

PLUS POINTS

+ Protects knees and joints of runners from damage by providing essential fatty acids that are anti-inflammatory.

+ High protein content makes them an excellent training snack for muscle-building sports.

+ Anti-oestrogen effect of linseed may help reduce PMS symptoms that can disrupt exercise routines.

sunflower seeds

These are a good source of iron, zinc and vitamin C; they are rich in polyunsaturated oil and used to make sunflower oil. The seeds are flat and oval-shaped, with a distinctive black striped shell. Once shelled, they can be nibbled as a snack or added to cakes, biscuits, bread and other baked products. They are a popular ingredient in cereal bars and in savoury vegetarian dishes. Add to stir-fries, rice dishes and pasta. Toasted, they may be tossed over fruit salads.

linseed

This is the seed of the flax plant. It is added to cereals and breads and sold in health food shops because the oils in the seeds are rich in omega-3 fatty acids, which protect against heart disease, and lignans (beneficial plant hormones with antioxidant activity, see opposite). It is also eaten as a means of adding bulk to the diet.

bone up on calciume

We need a good, lifelong supply of calcium for strong healthy bones and teeth and, in particular, to prevent osteoporosis (demineralization of bones, which can lead to fractures and breaks later in life). Apart from dairy foods and eggs, good sources of calcium include wholegrain cereals, muesli, oatmeal, pulses, nuts and seeds (for example, sesame seeds and sesame paste – tahini), dark green vegetables and dried fruit.

pumpkin seeds

These large seeds are flat and oval with a whitish shell. They are a rich source of iron and zinc, and are available from health food shops and supermarkets, usually shelled if bought in the latter. They can be roasted before eating as a snack or adding to salads, muesli and other breakfast cereal and vegetarian savoury dishes. Use also as a topping for breads and biscuits and as an ingredient in granola bars and flapjack-style slices.

sesame seeds

These are small flat cream-coloured seeds (brown ones are available in oriental stores). They are rich in unsaturated oils and calcium, plus vitamin E and minerals. They are familiar as the topping to prawn toasts in Chinese cuisine and as an addition to snack bars and confectionery. Sesame seeds can be eaten roasted or raw. Mix them with breadcrumbs for coating food before frying. Sesame seed paste is called tahini. It is used as a spread in the Middle East, and as an ingredient it forms the basis of two famous recipes: hummus (savoury) and halva (sweet).

Sesame seeds are also pressed (after roasting) to make sesame oil, which has a rich flavour and is used in stir-fries and other oriental recipes.

lignans

Lignans are similar to isoflavones (see page 125) but have so far been poorly researched. They are found primarily in linseeds, which contain 675-808 mcg per 100 g (3½ oz) of food. Flour ground from the seeds contains a little less, at 527 mcg per 100 g (3½ oz). Other food sources include lentils with around 18 mcg, which seems a minute amount compared with linseeds but is still a useful source. Other grains contain lignans: per 100 g (3½ oz), oat bran has 7 mcg, rye 6 mcg, wheat 5 mcg. Carrots contain around 4 mcg and asparagus 3 mcg.

seeds as a source of protein

Protein in foods is made up of amino acids (protein building blocks). In meat, fish, dairy food and eggs, the eight essential amino acids that cannot be made in the body are available in the right proportion. However, none of the three plant protein food groups supplies all eight essential amino acids. This means that a vegetarian diet should combine foods from at least two of the three groups to obtain the correct balance of amino acids, although they need not be eaten at the same meal:

- nuts and seeds
- pulses (beans including soy beans, chickpeas, lentils)
- grains (rice, bread, pasta and other wheat products, rye, barley, oats)

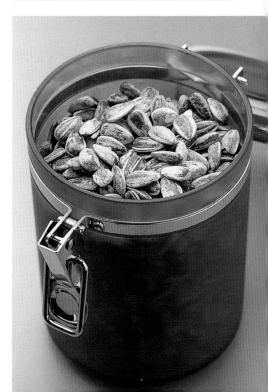

panforte

Panforte is eaten in small servings because it is rich, and packed with energy. Adding seeds to the traditional dried fruit and nut mixture increases the nutritional value.

preparation time **20–25 minutes**
cooking time **45 minutes**
serves **20**

100 g (3½ oz) skinned hazelnuts
100 g (3½ oz) skinned almonds
50 g (2 oz) sunflower seeds, lightly toasted
50 g (2 oz) pine nuts, lightly toasted
200 g (7 oz) pack candied fruit (orange, lemon, citron/melon), chopped
100 g (3½ oz) candied peel
2 teaspoons ground cinnamon
½ teaspoon ground nutmeg
½ teaspoon ground cloves or allspice
125 g (4 oz) unbleached plain flour
150 g (5 oz) clear honey
150 g (5 oz) brown sugar

1 Line the base and sides of a 20 cm (8 inch) square or round cake tin with rice paper.
2 Lightly toast the chopped nuts and seeds under the grill, turning several times. Alternatively, bake the seeds for about 10–15 minutes, turning until lightly golden. Or toast in a pan until evenly coloured.
3 Mix together the nuts, seeds, fruit, peel, spices and flour.
4 Warm the honey and sugar in a saucepan or in a jug in a microwave oven until the sugar dissolves, then add to the dry ingredients and bind with the honey mixture. Press into the lined tin and top with another layer of rice paper. Press down lightly.
5 Bake in a preheated oven, 150°C (300°F), Gas Mark 2, for 30 minutes. Remove from the oven and cool completely before cutting. The panforte can be stored in an airtight tin for up to 2 weeks.

golden muffins

Linseeds (or flaxseeds) are added to the muffin mixture and also used as decoration. The saffron, dried pear and mango enhance the golden colour and give a unique flavour.

preparation time **15 minutes**
cooking time **20–25 minutes**
makes **10**

175 g (6 oz) organic plain white flour
2 teaspoons baking powder
50 g (2 oz) golden caster sugar
3 large dried pears, diced
75 g (3 oz) dried mango, diced
4–5 tablespoons golden linseeds
pinch of saffron threads
2 tablespoons warm milk
50 g (2 oz) butter or margarine
1 free-range egg
1 teaspoon vanilla essence
300 ml (½ pint) carton buttermilk

1 Line a muffin pan with 10 paper cases or lightly oil the cups.
2 Sift the flour into a mixing bowl with the baking powder. Stir in the sugar, pears, mango and 3 tablespoons of the linseeds.
3 Infuse the saffron in the warm milk for 10 minutes.
4 Melt the butter or margarine and allow to cool.
5 Lightly beat together the egg and vanilla and stir into the buttermilk with the cooled melted butter.
6 Fold the egg mixture into the dry ingredients then spoon the mixture into the paper cases and sprinkle over the remaining seeds (you may need only 1½ tablespoons). Bake in a preheated oven, 190°C (375°F), Gas Mark 5, for 20–25 minutes, or until a skewer inserted in the centre comes out clean.
7 Leave to cool. The muffins will keep in an airtight container for up to 2 days, or can be frozen.

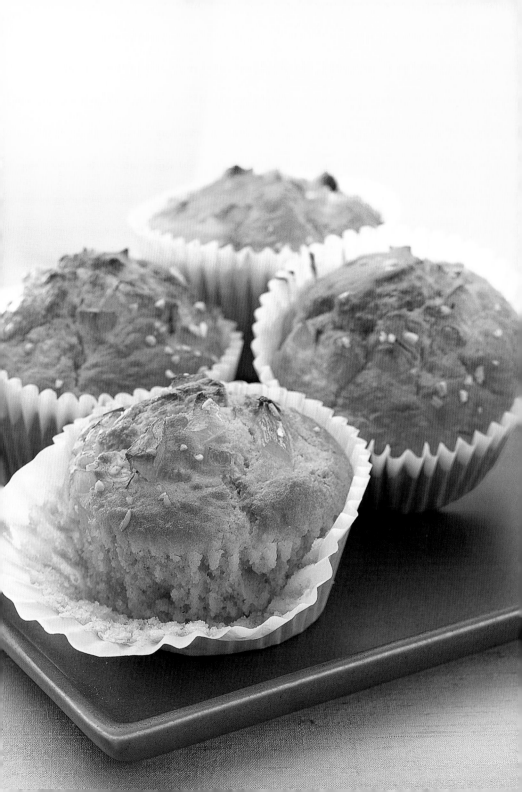

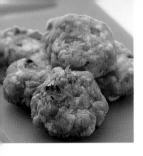

pork

Pork can be one of the leanest meats and yet it is often overlooked by those considering healthy eating. It is also versatile, being equally at home – and delicious – in both eastern and western cooking and can be used as an ingredient in burgers, meatballs, for stuffing vegetables and in cottage-pie-style dishes, pasta sauces, kebabs and stir-fries.

POWER CONTENT

Vitamin B1 and B6
Iron
Zinc
Amino acids
High in unsaturated fats

PLUS POINTS

+ Great source of selenium and zinc, vital antioxidants that protect against cell damage during aerobic activities.

+ Selenium and zinc also assist in wound-healing and recovery from injuries.

+ High protein content makes them an excellent training snack for muscle building sports.

Pork can be one of the highest-fat meat dishes – for example, roast pork with crackling. But lean pork is among the least fatty meats. The composition of extra lean pork is also lower in fat than equivalent red meats such as beef and lamb.

great for minerals

Lean pork is an excellent source of selenium, typically containing 13 mcg per 100 g (3½ oz) compared with only 3 mcg for lean beef and 1 mcg for lean lamb. Pork, like other meat, also provides the minerals iron and zinc (more than poultry and fish, but less than red meat), and it also contains magnesium, which is needed for growth, healthy bones and skin. Selenium and zinc are both powerful antioxidants, helping to protect the body's DNA from damage by free radicals.

Although pork does not contain as much iron as redder meats, it still contains enough to help prevent the symptoms of tiredness and ultimately anaemia.

meat for strength

Protein is needed not just for children and adolescents, but for all ages. However, the idea that meat protein is superior to vegetarian protein is now regarded as old-fashioned. A vegetarian diet can be every bit as healthy as a non-vegetarian one (conversely, it is perfectly possible to eat an unhealthy vegetarian diet). However, meat does contain all the amino acids (building blocks of protein) in the right proportions for muscle growth and tissue repair, while vegetable proteins must be eaten in certain combinations during the day for maximum benefit (see Seeds, pages 100–101).

how much meat?

Two daily portions of meat are adequate for everyone except very active, fast-growing adolescents. For a guide to portions and more about eating meat, see page 19.

Suggestions that eating meat can increase the risk of cancer of the colon are still being investigated. However, epidemiological studies comparing diet with incidence of disease correlate a high intake of vegetables, fruit and starchy foods with a lower incidence of cancer, so we should, in any case, eat lots of vegetables with our meat, for their antioxidant protection.

make it lean mince

Mince is meat that has been ground or minced, and the fat content will vary depending on the cuts of meat and fat included. Generally it will be quite high in fat. EU regulations stipulate the fat content of mince, which varies with different meats. In the case of standard pork mince, the upper limit is 30 per cent, which is quite high. For that reason it is important to buy pork mince labelled as 'lean', which must not contain more than 7 per cent fat. 'Extra lean' pork mince contains even less fat, usually below 5 per cent, although supermarkets have their own grading system.

boost your B vitamins

Pork contains more B vitamins than other red meat and has a particularly high vitamin B1 (thiamin) content. Thiamin is needed to transmit messages between brain and spinal cord, and it is also essential for enzymes that convert food into fuel for the body. In addition, pork is rich in vitamin B6, which is important in protein metabolism, and for healthy skin and nerves. It is also needed for the formation of antibodies (which help fight infection) and for the formation of haemoglobin which transports oxygen around the body in red blood cells.

Zinc is vital for male fertility and is thought to work together with selenium to increase both the number and mobility of healthy sperm.

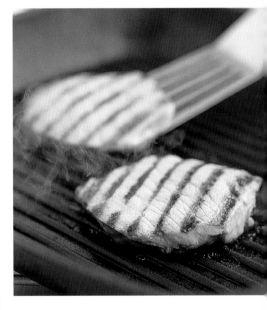

the organic option

Organic pork (and other organic meat) is produced by a system of farming that does not use growth promoters and other prophylactic drugs, such as antibiotics, as a matter of routine. Agrochemicals such as pesticides are not used and the livestock is fed an organic diet. Often the animals are fed on grass (as opposed to recycled animal protein and other artificial feed), which means that the meat has a more healthy fat profile with a greater proportion of unsaturated to saturated fats. Organic livestock also enjoy higher standards of animal welfare, in terms of space and free-range facilities, than non-organic livestock.

pork kofte kebabs

This mix can also be used to make home-made burgers, and you can vary the meat (and herbs and spices) to suit your taste: chicken, beef and lamb also work very well.

preparation time **10 minutes**
cooking time **20 minutes**
serves **4**

250 g (8 oz) ground lean (less than
   5 per cent fat) pork
1 large onion, quartered
1 garlic clove, peeled and halved
1 chilli, cored and deseeded
2 teaspoons tomato purée
15 g (½ oz) coriander leaves
15 g (½ oz) parsley leaves
sea salt and freshly ground black pepper

1 Put all the ingredients into a food processor or mixing bowl and combine well.

2 Divide the meat paste into quarters and form around 4 skewers. Cover the kebabs and refrigerate until they are needed.

3 When ready to cook, lift the kebabs carefully on to a grill pan lined with foil that has been brushed with oil to prevent sticking during cooking.

4 Grill under a preheated moderately hot grill for 15–20 minutes, turning several times until the kebabs have browned on the outside and are thoroughly cooked through. Serve with Tabbouleh (page 86) and a green salad.

pork stir-fry

Stir-fries are one of the tastiest ways to eat vegetables. They also allow a moderate amount of meat to go a long way.

preparation time **15 minutes**
cooking time **15 minutes**
serves **4**

2 tablespoons vegetable oil
2 garlic cloves, finely chopped
1 teaspoon grated fresh root ginger
1 chilli, deseeded and diced
1 red pepper, cored, deseeded and cut into strips
3 carrots, cut into strips
1 large onion, sliced
250 g (8 oz) lean (less than 5 per cent fat)
   pork, cubed
1 courgette, sliced
1 small broccoli head, divided into florets
FOR THE SAUCE
2 tablespoons soy sauce
2 tablespoons orange juice
1 teaspoon tomato purée
1 teaspoon vinegar
1 teaspoon demerara sugar

1 Heat the oil in a wok or large frying pan and add the garlic, ginger and chilli to heat through but do not allow to colour.

2 Add the pepper, carrots, onion and pork and stir-fry over a moderate to high heat for about 5 minutes.

3 Add the courgette and broccoli and continue to stir-fry for a further 5 minutes.

4 Stir in the ingredients for the sauce and allow to bubble in the base of the wok, then toss the ingredients through the liquid as you stir-fry for a few more minutes.

5 Serve with steamed or boiled fragrant Thai rice. Ring the changes by serving with brown rice on occasion.

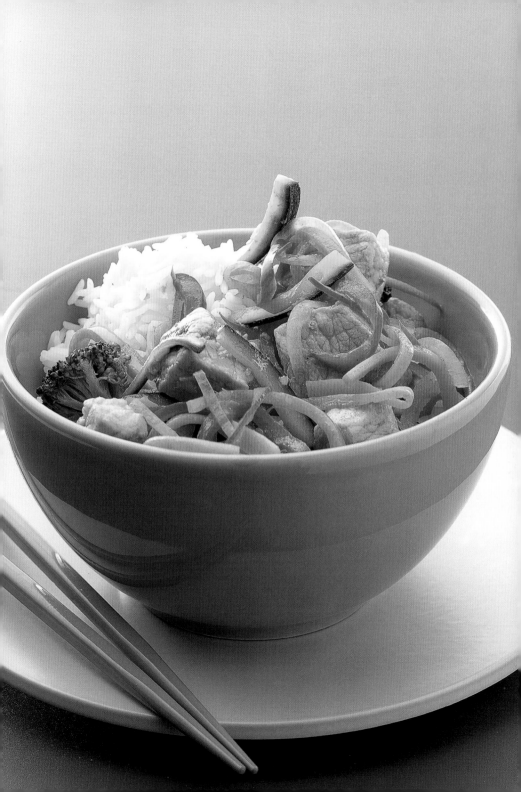

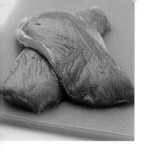

lean meat & game

Lean meat is an excellent concentrated source of protein for growth and repair in the body. It is rich in important vitamins and minerals – just don't overdo it, and partner it with lots of vegetables.

POWER CONTENT

B vitamins
Chromium
Iron
Magnesium
Potassium
Zinc

PLUS POINTS

+ You don't have to exist on steak to build muscle (as used to be thought), but lean red meat is a concentrated source of protein for body building and repair.

+ Lean meat is also rich in iron and other minerals that prevent tiredness and enable red blood cells to carry oxygen required for aerobic activity.

+ As a contributor of chromium, lean red meat helps the body regulate insulin and therefore blood sugar levels, vital for fuelling all physical activities.

Quantity and quality are the watchwords when thinking about eating meat, in terms of both your health and your finances. You can eat whatever type of meat you enjoy the most – so long as it is lean. While meat can be nutritious, it contains a lot of fat, especially saturated fat. Meat eaters get a hefty whack of their fat intake from meat products, which accounts for 25 per cent of fat in a typical diet.

So in order to eat meat, not fat, you are advised to avoid eating fatty meat and associated products. These include sausages, salami, pâté, meat pies and pastes, burgers, koftas, keemas and bacon. If avoiding these seems too hard, try just to use them very sparingly to flavour a dish.

keeping the fat down

Game is leaner than most red meats and even duck can be enjoyed if the fat is drained off during cooking (as in Peking duck) or the layer of fat and skin is removed from duck breasts either before or after cooking. Removing skin from other poultry also reduces the fat content. True game, such as venison and game birds like partridge and wild (not farmed) pheasant, grouse and woodcock also have a healthier fat profile. This is because they exercise more than farmed birds that are reared mainly for shooting. The result is that their meat contains mainly mono-saturated and unsaturated fats instead of the saturated fats of intensively reared livestock. For this reason,

Lean red meat is an excellent source of chromium, which allows us to tolerate sugar and maintain blood-sugar levels. It also boosts the immune system and keeps brain transmitters healthy.

free-range and organic meat is also preferred, although not all of it is particularly energetic during its lifetime. However, the likelihood of residues of growth promoters, hormones and antibiotics is far lower in free-range products and should be all but absent in organic meat, which is produced by a system that does not allow use of the majority of agrochemicals and drugs for livestock. To benefit from the iron and other nutrients, choose the leanest.

nutrition and health

Meat provides in the correct proportions the eight amino acids necessary for growth and is also an excellent source of iron. As a rough guide the redder the meat, the more iron it contains. In this respect, red meat means not only beef and lamb, but also pork, duck, venison, rabbit and the myriad game birds, such as pheasant, partridge, grouse and others available throughout the game calendar.

Red meat and game are also excellent sources of zinc, which is needed for preventing anaemia and related tiredness as well as for reproductive health, particularly in men.

Chromium is not a mineral that we hear much about, but lean red meat is a good source, and it is vital in one particular area – namely how the body tolerates sugar and handles blood-sugar levels, because chromium is essential for insulin activity. It also has a chemical role, along with other substances, in reducing blood fat levels and increasing the concentration of beneficial HDL cholesterol. In addition, it is involved in immune responses and brain-nerve transmitters. A truly powerful nutrient!

Meat also provides that vital antioxidant mineral selenium, plus another with an antioxidant role, copper; also phosphorus for bones, potassium to counterbalance sodium and help regulate blood pressure, and magnesium. Like chromium, magnesium is a mineral bound up in many body functions,

avoid the burnt bits

Char-grilling may be fashionable, but charred and burnt bits that form on the surface of meat cooked by grilling, roasting, frying and barbecuing contain substances (heterocyclic amines) that have provoked cancer in animal feed trials and damaged human DNA in test tube studies. You can be a fast or slow metabolizer of these substances, a factor that is determined genetically. It seems that individuals with the fast type of enzyme system are at increased risk of developing polyps and large bowel cancer. Research in this area continues, and it is probably best for everyone to avoid the burnt bits.

including helping the B vitamins work well and stabilizing calcium in the body for strong bones and teeth. It also similarly helps with nerve impulses and is necessary for heart health.

Another nutrient in good supply in red meat is the B group of vitamins, particularly vitamins B1 (thiamin), B2 (riboflavin) and B3 (niacin), B6 (pyridoxine) and B12 – all essential for the body to run smoothly.

what is a serving of meat?

Two daily portions of meat are adequate for most people, although very active sportspeople, and adolescents during growth spurts, may have a third. For more details, see page 19.

eat less meat to protect your gut bacteria

The amount of meat you eat influences the bacteria that live in your gut to ferment undigested food residues to produce healthy – or toxic – by-products. Heavy meat consumption increases the proportion of harmful bacteria that produce potential toxins.

peppered steaks
with spinach mash

preparation time **20 minutes**
cooking time **25 minutes**
serves **4**

750 g (1½ lb) potatoes, peeled and chopped
250 g (8 oz) fresh spinach leaves
3 tablespoons extra virgin olive oil
1½ tablespoons lemon juice
4 beef medallions, about 125–150 g (4–5 oz) each
2 tablespoons cracked black peppercorns
150 ml (¼ pint) red wine
1½ tablespoons redcurrant jelly
2 tablespoons red wine vinegar

1 Boil the potatoes until tender. Drain, reserving
   50 ml (2 fl oz) of the cooking water. Keep the
   potatoes covered in a pan with the reserved water.
2 Wash the spinach and put it in a pan without any
   extra water. Cover and cook for 3–4 minutes. Drain.
3 Mash the potatoes with the reserved water, 2
   tablespoons of the olive oil and the lemon juice.
   Season to taste and stir the spinach lightly into the
   mash to give a thick marbling effect. Keep warm.
4 Meanwhile, prepare the meat. Place the cracked
   peppercorns on a plate and press both sides of the
   steaks on to the pepper to cover them. Brush the
   steaks with a little oil, sprinkle with a little salt and
   cook on a preheated griddle or in a heavy-based
   frying pan for 3–4 minutes on each side. The steaks
   should be browned on the outside but still pink in
   the middle.
5 Remove the steaks, add the wine to the pan and
   bring to the boil. Add the redcurrant jelly and vinegar
   and boil rapidly for 5 minutes, or until the liquid has
   reduced by half.
6 To serve, put each steak on a warmed plate, pour
   over some of the red wine jus and place some
   spinach mash alongside.

juicy burgers

Home-made burgers using lean red meat need
not be fatty, especially if they are grilled and served
with a mixed salad and healthy homemade chips
(see page 61).

preparation time **15 minutes**
cooking time **about 16 minutes**
serves **4**

500 g (1 lb) lean or low-fat minced lamb or beef
2 carrots, grated
3 teaspoons tomato purée
2 tablespoons chopped parsley
vegetable oil, for frying
4 burger buns
salt and freshly ground black pepper
TO GARNISH
crispy lettuce
sliced tomatoes
onions, cut into rings
TO SERVE
mustard or other relishes

1 Mix the meat, carrot, tomato purée and parsley in
   a bowl with the seasoning.
2 Shape the mixture into 4 burgers.
3 Lightly oil a frying pan and then cook the burgers
   for about 8 minutes on each side. For lower-fat
   cooking, grill under a medium-high heat for the
   same length of time.
4 Slice each burger bun in half horizontally. Place a
   layer of lettuce on the base of the unspread bun,
   and put the burger on top. Add the tomatoes and
   onion and cover with the top of the bun.

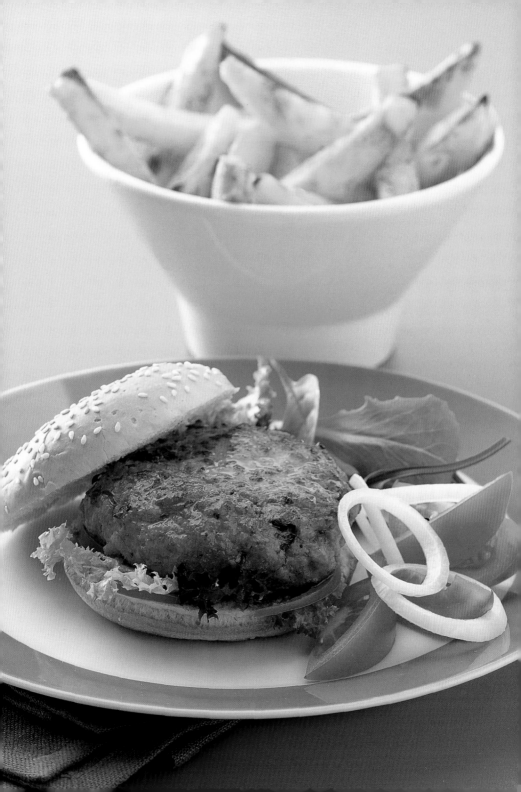

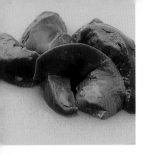

liver

Liver might have been an aphrodisiac to the Romans, but it does not turn on many people these days, which is a shame, because it is a very nutritious food and can be extremely appetizing – even for people who think they are not going to like it.

POWER CONTENT

Vitamin A
Vitamin B1, B2, B6 and B12
Iron
Protein
Zinc

PLUS POINTS

+ Rich source of iron to help prevent the lack of energy that is related to anaemia.

+ Excellent source of selenium, a valuable antioxidant that makes enzymes that protect against free-radical damage.

+ Contains copper and other minerals to boost immunity and offset any side-effects of too much physical activity.

masses of minerals

Liver is an excellent source of the trace elements iron, zinc, selenium and copper. Selenium is a valuable antioxidant, providing protection for the body's cells. It works with vitamin E and helps maintain the body's immune system. It is a component of many enzymes needed for running body functions and is the subject of many studies designed to assess its potential as an anti-cancer nutrient.

Zinc is an important component of many enzymes, including superoxide dismutase (a powerful antioxidant enzyme that neutralizes potentially damaging free radicals). Eating liver, which is rich in copper, iron and zinc, also aids growth of hair, skin and nails and boosts immune cell function.

not for pregnant women

Due to intensive animal feed being used in modern farming, a government health warning advises pregnant women not to eat liver. It contains high levels of vitamin A, which could induce developmental abnormalities in a foetus, particularly in the early stages of pregnancy. This is a pity, because liver is one of the richest sources of folates. For the same reason, vitamin A supplements should not be taken in pregnancy. Vitamin A in excess is always dangerous because it is fat-soluble, so the body stores it rather than excreting excess, as happens with water-soluble vitamins such as B and C.

Lamb's liver is nutritionally superior to both chicken and calves' liver, but all sources are good.

vital vitamins

Vitamin A needed for healthy skin structure and mucus-secreting tissues; for eyesight, particularly night vision; healthy skin and growth in children. WARNING Too much vitamin A during pregnancy can be problematic (see box left).

Vitamin B1 (thiamin) needed to transmit messages between brain and spinal cord. Vital for enzymes that convert food into fuel.

Vitamin B2 (riboflavin) makes energy available in the body. Works with vitamin B6, folic acid and iron and promotes skin and eye health.

Vitamin B6 (pyridoxine) key in protein metabolism. Promotes healthy skin and is essential for the nervous system. Also needed for the formation of haemoglobin in red blood cells and of antibodies to fight infection.

Vitamin B12 liver contains the highest amounts of this vitamin of any meat. Essential for synthesis of DNA, the basis of body cell production, particularly of red blood cells that are needed for transporting iron in the blood. Deficiency leads to anaemia. Also maintains the myelin sheath, a layer of insulation round the nerves, so deficiency will damage nerves.

thanks for the memory

Memory-enhancing nutrients are found in abundance in liver: B vitamins and choline. The latter is not a true vitamin, which is loosely defined as a substance that the body cannot make. Choline may be synthesized in the liver. It is regarded as a member of the B vitamin complex and is associated with lecithin, a natural emulsifier that keeps fats in suspension. Choline concentrates in the brain and has a function in memory formation and brain function.

how much liver?

Although liver is very nutritious in many respects, it does contain two or three times the amount of cholesterol compared with muscle meat. For this reason, it is often avoided by some health-conscious people. In so doing, they overlook the fact that a greater proportion of the total fat in liver is of polyunsaturated fats than in lean muscle meat. There is absolutely no harm – and there are many benefits – in eating liver once a week, which is probably often enough even for fans, especially when there are so many other foods to enjoy in a varied diet. A portion of liver is about 3 medium pieces, enough for one meal.

country style liver pâté

A low-fat version of this popular retro recipe.

preparation time **15 minutes**
cooking time **50 minutes**
serves **8**

6 rashers of lean back bacon, smoked or
   unsmoked
2 onions, roughly chopped
2 garlic cloves, roughly chopped
250 g (8 oz) chopped lean pork
250 g (8 oz) lamb's liver
15 g (½ oz) flat leaf parsley
2 cloves
1 small piece of mace
a grating of nutmeg
100 ml (3½ fl oz) red wine

1 Flatten the bacon rashers using the blade of a
palette knife, and use to line a buttered ovenproof
terrine of 600 ml (1 pint) capacity.
2 Put the onions, garlic, pork, liver and parsley into a
food processor and chop roughly.
3 Crush the cloves and mace using a pestle and
mortar, and add to the mixture with the nutmeg.
4 Add the wine and carefully combine, then pour into
the prepared terrine. Stand the terrine in a dish of
hot water and bake in a preheated oven, 180°C
(350°F), Gas Mark 4, for 50 minutes.
5 Remove from the oven and leave to stand until
completely cold. Invert the terrine over a plate to
remove the pâté, then cover and store in the
refrigerator until needed. Serve with green salad,
tomato salad and lots of hot crusty bread or toast.

quick liver one-pot

Liver is one of those things you love or hate
– lovers of liver have a nutritional advantage
and they will find this recipe extremely easy to
make and very tasty.

preparation time **15 minutes**
cooking time **20 minutes**
serves **4**

1 tablespoon olive oil
2 onions, sliced
3 carrots, cut into ribbons
4 rashers of lean back bacon
1 tablespoon redcurrant jelly
1 tablespoon tomato purée
500 g (1 lb) lamb's liver
sea salt and freshly ground black pepper

1 Heat the oil in a heavy-based saucepan with a
well-fitting lid. Add the onion, carrot and bacon
and cook over a low heat for 10 minutes, stirring
occasionally.
2 Add the redcurrant jelly and tomato purée and cook
for a further 2 minutes, stirring a couple of times.
3 Add the liver, cover the pan and leave to cook for
about 5 minutes, then stir to mix all the ingredients
well. Season, replace the lid, and cook for a further
2–3 minutes. Serve immediately, with mashed
potatoes and a selection of green vegetables, such
as cabbage, green beans, peas or Brussels sprouts.

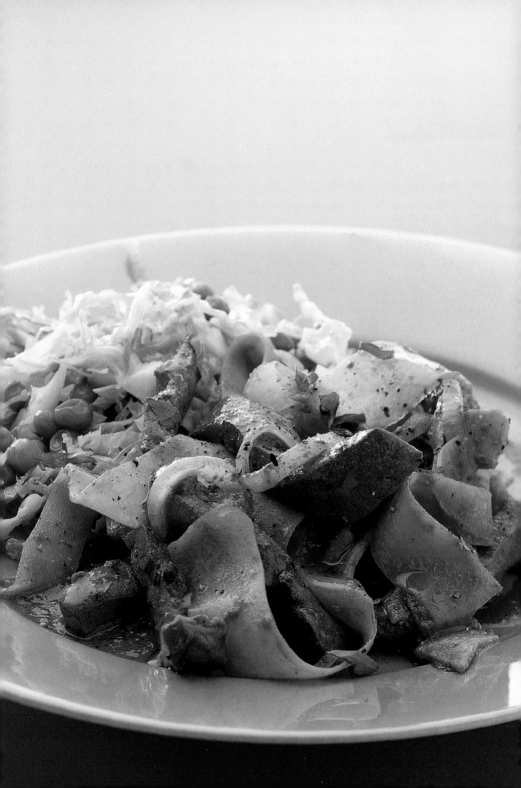

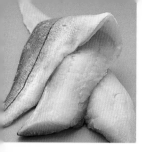

fish

Fish is one of the quickest and easiest low-fat, high-protein foods to prepare. It is an important part of a healthy everyday diet and is especially easy to use as there is so much variety within the food group; white fish is very low in fat and full of minerals and oily fish is a vital provider of the essential omega-3 fatty acids.

POWER CONTENT

Vitamin A
Vitamin D
Calcium
Fluoride
Phosphorus
Protein
Omega-3 fatty acids

PLUS POINTS

+ **Excellent source of protein for muscle-building and body repairs.**

+ **Oily fish provide more calories than white fish for fuelling endurance activities, and the oils from these extra calories are the beneficial unsaturated ones.**

+ **Iodine in fish is essential for regulating hormone production that controls all body functions to enable fitness.**

Fish is similar to seafood in that on its own it can be a very low fat meal, however, there is a tendency to add a creamy sauce which immediately piles on the fat. Stick to cooking white and oily fish as simply as possible – a little lemon juice and black pepper often tastes the best.

varieties of oily fish

Most salmon is farmed, but small amounts of wild and organic salmon are available. This is paler, leaner and firmer because the flesh has not been coloured with (natural) dyes added to its food and it has exercised more than farmed fish.

Salmon trout is a name used to describe either very large rainbow trout or sea-grown rainbow trout. Rainbow trout is the main breed of farmed trout. It originated in North American lakes and streams and is

the benefits of fish

All types of fish are an excellent low-fat protein food. White fish (e.g. cod, haddock, and plaice) is especially low in fat and rich in minerals, including iodine. Iodine is also found in seafood and oily fish. It comes from sea plants eaten by fish and is necessary in humans to prevent goitre and for production of the thyroid hormone thyroxine.

recognizable by a broad purple or violet band along the flanks and black spots on the tail fin. Brown trout is the native European freshwater trout. The colour varies, but is usually brownish with black and rusty red spots – saltwater versions are known as sea trout.

Herring, mackerel, sardine and shad are all types of oily fish which have soft flesh.

omega-3 oils in fish

Oily fish have the advantage of being rich in essential polyunsaturates called omega-3 fatty acids. Omega-3 oils make the blood less sticky and therefore less likely to clot and cause a heart attack. They also help reduce blood pressure. Some omega-3 oil survives canning. Canned fish (e.g. sardines, pilchards) are rich in calcium, phosphorus and fluoride because the bones are edible; boned canned fish is therefore nutritionally inferior. In addition, oily fish contains the fat-soluble vitamins A and D.

how much to eat

To be of benefit, fish needs to be a regular part of the diet. Eating two fish meals a week, and making one of the meals oily fish, will give you the right amount of omega-3 fats for health. Fish also contains unsaturated fats and contributes to a lower fat intake.

buying fish

Allow 150 g (5 oz) per person for steaks and fillets and cutlets and 375 g (12 oz) for whole fish on the bone. Fresh fish is best used on the day it is bought, but it will keep in the refrigerator at 4°C (40°F) for up to 3 days. Pre-packed fresh fish will probably keep longer because the packs are flushed with a mixture of gases that slow down bacterial growth. If the fish has not been previously frozen it can safely be frozen at home; previously frozen fish is unsuitable for freezing. For best results freeze fish that is as fresh as possible; this is why frozen-at-sea fish is usually the best.

typical omega-3 fatty acid content of fish

Food	Average portion (g)	Total omega-3g/100g food per portion
• Cod	120	0.30
• Haddock	120	0.19
• Plaice	130	0.42
• Herring	119	2.18
• Mackerel	160	4.46
• Pilchards, canned in tomato sauce	110	3.16
• Sardines, canned in tomato sauce	100	2.02
• Salmon, canned in brine	100	1.85
• Salmon	100	2.5
• Trout	230	2.92
• Prawns, frozen raw	60	0.91
• Cod liver oil	5ml/1 tsp	1.19

Omega-3 Fatty Acids and Health report, British Nutrition Foundation

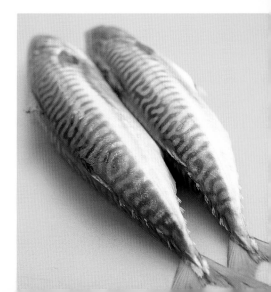

mackerel pâté

The secret of this pâté is the use of mace, which has a unique flavour and enhances that of the fish. Try to buy the highest quality mace you can find; the redder in colour the better the quality.

preparation time **15 minutes**
serves **4**

2 smoked mackerel fillets, skinned
1 generous blade of mace
75 g (3 oz) unsalted butter
250 g (8 oz) low-fat soft white cheese
juice of 1 lemon
grated rind of ½ lemon
freshly ground black pepper
TO SERVE
selection of crudités (raw vegetables), such as
    carrots, radicchio, celery, cucumber, peppers,
    spring onions, chicory leaves

1 Flake the fish into a food processor.
2 Pound the mace with a pestle in a mortar, then add to the mackerel.
3 Beat the butter to soften and add to the food processor, together with the cheese, lemon juice and rind. Blend to a thick purée.
4 Season to taste with black pepper. Serve with the crudités and hot thinly sliced wholemeal toast.

goan-style fish stew

The coastal strip of Goa in southern India is famous for its seafood and green fish curries. This approximation can be made using any types of fish, and is a particularly tasty way of eating more oily fish.

preparation time **30 minutes**
cooking time **30 minutes**
serves **4**

1 garlic clove, crushed
2.5 cm (1 inch) fresh root ginger, peeled and grated
1 onion, chopped
1 teaspoon ground coriander
1 teaspoon ground cumin
¼ teaspoon ground turmeric
3 tablespoons sunflower oil
4 tomatoes, skinned and chopped
50 g (2 oz) creamed coconut, grated
300 ml (½ pint) boiling water
400 g (13 oz) coley, cut into chunks
400 g (13 oz) mackerel fillets, skinned
250 g (8 oz) spinach leaves
3 tablespoons chopped fresh coriander
sea salt and freshly ground pepper

1 Sauté the garlic, ginger, onion and spices in the oil for 10 minutes, being careful not to let them brown.
2 Add the tomatoes, cover and cook for a further 10 minutes.
3 Dissolve the creamed coconut in the water and stir into the tomato mixture. Add the fish and the spinach and cook gently for 8 minutes.
4 Stir in the fresh coriander and continue to cook for another couple of minutes, then season to taste. Serve with rice or naan breads.

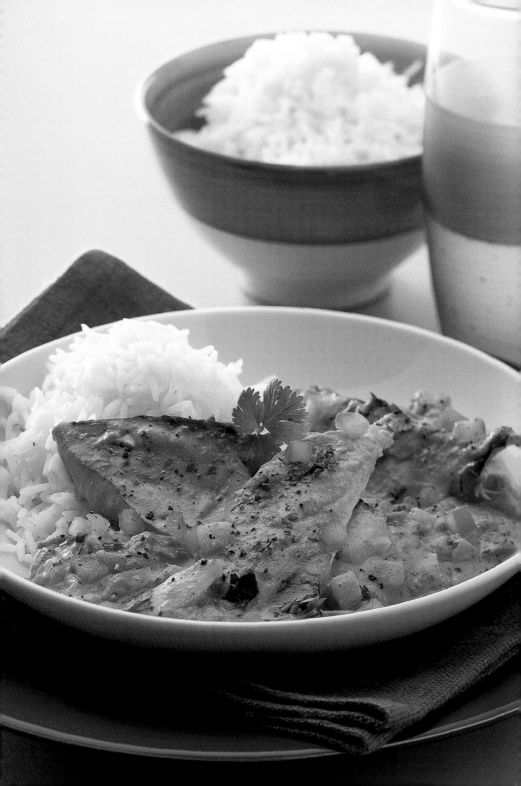

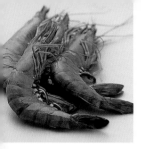

seafood

Seafood describes both fish and shellfish. The special value of oily fish is described on pages 116–117. Seafood includes oysters, mussels, crabs, clams and scallops, all of which are invaluable for their unique flavours and rich mineral content.

POWER CONTENT

Scallops
Calcium
Phosphorus
Potassium
Iron
Zinc

Prawns
Calcium
Iron
Phosphorus
Zinc
Carotenes

PLUS POINTS

+ A fantastic low-fat provider of protein for those who need concentrated sources for their sports activities.

+ Rich in calcium, phosphorus, iron, zinc and other minerals needed to produce antioxidant enzymes that protect against the effects of physical stress.

+ A body-building food that is a good source of potassium.

Seafood gained an undeserved bad nutritional reputation in the 1980s, when early nutritional analysis revealed lobster to have high sterol levels. From this it was assumed that lobster had high cholesterol levels, and the bad news that seafood contained too much cholesterol stuck. Later, more sophisticated analyses showed that only a small proportion of the sterols were cholesterol and that the majority were benign, even beneficial. Nutritionally, a lobster is in the same cholesterol league as a trout or a flounder – in other words, the fat content is not a problem. Indeed, seafood is as beneficial a low-fat protein food as fish.

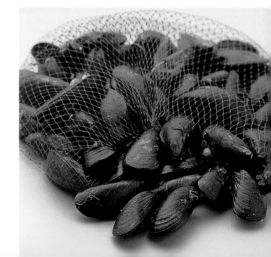

Seafood is far lower in fat than many so-called
healthy eating foods containing less than 5 per cent
fat per average portion.

genuine low-fat food

Seafood is far lower in fat than many so-called healthy
eating foods – for example, biscuits, bars and crisps
that claim to be 85 per cent fat-free do actually contain
15 per cent fat. To be a true low-fat food, a food has to
contain 5 per cent fat or less, a category into which
seafood fits very comfortably in its raw state. So eating
seafood regularly can help lower fat intake. The trick is
to prepare it without any or too much additional fat.
Dishes such as moules marinière are better than
moules à la bonne femme (in cream sauce). In
combination with whole grains and vegetables (peas,
broccoli), seafood has great potential in the heart-
healthy eating stakes. Giving preference to fresh fish
over salty breaded and crumbed processed fish will
increase potassium intake, a major step in reducing the
risk of rising blood pressure with age. And as this book
emphasizes, healthy eating is about enjoyment as well
as putting foods in proportion in the long term.

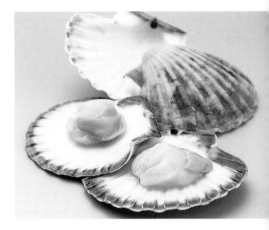

buying prawns and scallops

Seafood should be used as soon as possible, preferably
on the day it is bought. Do not keep it in the refrigerator
for more than a day.

Prawns can be bought live, but are usually sold
cooked and shelled. Live prawns are grey and turn pink
on cooking. There are various types of prawn, including
langoustines (also called scampi or Dublin Bay prawns),
large prawns and common prawns. Tiger prawns are
very large and are sometimes 'butterflied' (as are large
prawns and scampi). To do this, shell the prawn and
make a full-length cut along the inside curve, about
half-way through the flesh. Devein the prawn, then open
it out to a butterfly shape before cooking.

Opening scallops

Scallops are usually sold opened and cleaned, with the
intestines removed. If not, open by holding the shell,
rounded side uppermost, and inserting a short sharp
blade (such as an oyster knife) into the hinge muscle.
Twist the blade and pull back the rounded shell.
Discard the top shell. Scrape away the fringe and cut
out the black intestines, then slip the blade beneath
the scallop to remove it from the bottom shell. The
coral part should remain intact, as it is edible – in fact,
it is considered by many to be a delicacy.

alive alive oh –
with minerals galore

**Seafood is a rich source of protein and
minerals, and has a low fat content. Scallops
and prawns typically contain less than 1 per
cent fat. Prawns are notable for their calcium,
phosphorus, iron and zinc content. The pink
colouring of prawns is from the carotene
content of their shells – and carotenoids are a
valuable antioxidant, more so in food than as a
vitamin supplement. Scallops are curiously rich
in beneficial potassium and contain slightly
less of the same minerals as prawns, while the
greatest proportion of their minimal fat content
is polyunsaturated, including beneficial omega-
3 fats (see Fish, pages 116–117).**

oriental scallops with wild rice

Scallops are often cooked in rich sauces, but are equally suited to low-fat stir-frying. Their delicate flavour goes particularly well with nutty wild rice.

preparation time **15 minutes**
cooking time **45 minutes**
serves **4**

75 g (3 oz) wild rice
75 g (3 oz) brown rice
2 tablespoons sunflower oil
8 scallops, removed from the shell, halved
   horizontally and separated from the roe
1 tablespoon sesame oil
2 garlic cloves, chopped
1 teaspoon grated fresh root ginger
150 g (5 oz) shiitake mushrooms, sliced
1 bunch of spring onions, sliced
100 g (3½ oz) mange tout
1 tablespoon light soy sauce
sea salt and freshly ground black pepper

1 Boil the wild rice in plenty of water for about 40 minutes. Add the brown rice 25 minutes before the end of cooking.
2 Fifteen minutes before the rice is cooked, prepare the remaining ingredients. Heat 1 tablespoon of the sunflower oil in a wok and fry the scallops and the roe over a high heat for 1 minute each side. Remove from the pan and keep warm in a covered dish.
3 Add the remaining sunflower oil to the wok with the sesame oil. When it is hot add the garlic, ginger, mushrooms, onions and mange tout, and stir-fry for 2 minutes.
4 Add the soy sauce and seasoning and return the scallops and roe to the pan. Heat through for a further 2 minutes. Serve immediately with the rice.

haddock & prawn fish cakes

Replacing two meat meals a week with fish is an important part of a healthy diet. With delicious taste combinations such as the haddock and prawns in this recipe, this benefit becomes a positive treat.

preparation time **20 minutes**
cooking time **20 minutes**
serves **4**

375 g (12 oz) haddock
1 bay leaf
6 peppercorns
1 small pack of parsley, leaves chopped
   and stalks reserved
125 g (4 oz) prawns, shelled and defrosted
250 g (8 oz) potato, boiled and mashed
1 tablespoon vegetable oil
salt and freshly ground black pepper

1 Poach the haddock with the bay leaf, peppercorns and parsley stalks, in enough water to cover, for about 10 minutes. When cooked, remove the fish from the cooking liquid and flake the fish from the bones and skin. Discard the herbs.
2 Mix the flaked haddock, prawns, mashed potato and 1 tablespoon of the chopped parsley and season to taste. Form the mixture into 4 fish cakes.
3 Lightly fry the fishcakes in 1 tablespoon of oil in a frying pan for 8–10 minutes each side until golden. Remove from the pan and drain off any excess fat, if necessary, on kitchen paper. Serve with potatoes and carrots, peas or a green salad, garnished with the remaining parsley.

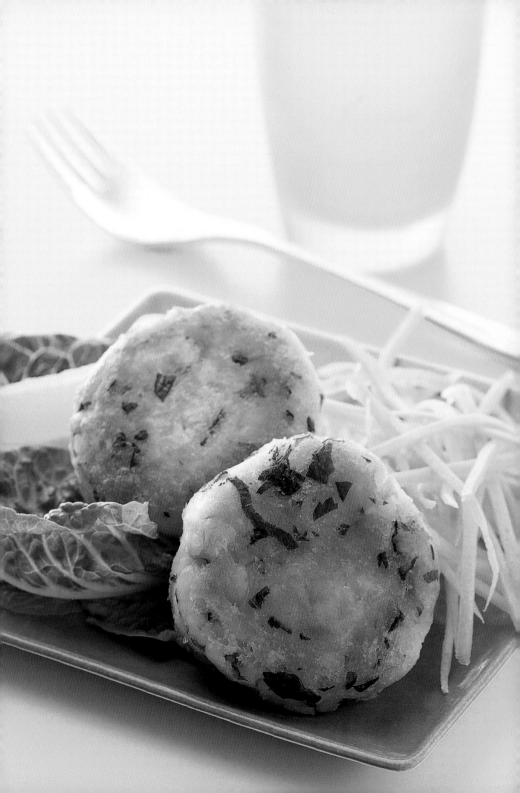

glossary

Alpha-Lipoic Acid An antioxidant enzyme.

Amino Acid The building blocks from which proteins are made. Technically speaking compounds of carbon, hydrogen, oxygen and nitrogen.

Amylose A type of starch in rice.

Amylopectin A type of starch in rice.

Antioxidants Vitamins, minerals, phytochemicals and other substances that protect against the damaging oxidative action of free radicals.

Beta-Carotene A pigment in orange, red and yellow foods that is turned into vitamin A in the body and also has antioxidant properties.

Bioflavonoids See flavonoids.

Biomass The living mass of bacteria that bulks up stools.

Blood Sugar Sugar in the blood derived from food and used by the body as fuel or energy.

Butyrate A by-product of bacterial fermentation in the gut that seems to protect against cancer.

Calcium A mineral for healthy bones and teeth.

Calorie A measure of energy.

Carbohydrate Simple or complex compounds in food; the major source of energy in the diet.

Carotenoids A group of orange, red and yellow pigments in food, including beta-carotene. Some have antioxidant properties.

Chlorophyll Green pigment present in plants that has antioxidant properties.

Cholesterol A fatty substance produced in the liver and transported in blood. Essential for many body functions, but a heart disease risk in excess.

Collagen Part of the structure of body tissues.

Diuretic A food or drink that increases the flow of urine.

DHA Docosahexaenoic acid, an omega-3 fatty acid found in fish oils.

EHA Eicosapentaenoic acid, an omega-3 fatty acid found in fish oils.

Ellagic Acid An antioxidant found in berries.

Endosperm The inner starchy part of a cereal grain.

Enzyme A protein that acts as a catalyst for metabolic reactions in the body.

Essential Fatty Acid Fats that are needed in the diet but which cannot be made by the body: linoleic acid, alpha-linolenic acid, arachidonic acid.

Fatty Acids Natural acids which are needed by the body for good health.

Fibre The non-digestible part of carbohydrate foods, either soluble or insoluble.

Flavonoid A group of between 3,500 and 4,000 substances in plant foods with antioxidant activities.

Folate The form in which a B vitamin essential for health is found in foods.

Folic Acid The synthetic form of folate found in vitamin supplements.

Free Radical A highly reactive substance found in the body and the environment (pollution, cigarette smoke) that triggers cancer and heart disease.

GLA Gamma-linolenic acid, produced by the omega-6 essential fatty acid linoleic acid. Production in the body can be blocked by too much saturated fat in the diet, too much alcohol and an imbalance of omega-3 and omega-6 intake.

Gluten Protein in wheat, rye, barley and oats.

GI Glycaemic index, which is the measure of the effect of food on blood sugar levels.

Haemoglobin Part of red blood cells that carries oxygen to the tissues.

HDL High density lipoprotein, a type of cholesterol that is beneficial.

Homocysteine Beneficial substance created in the body by the amino acid methionine.

Hormone Chemical secreted by the endocrine glands to regulate body functions.

Insulin Hormone produced in the pancreas to regulate blood sugar levels.

Iodine Trace element in seafood needed for the production of thyroid hormones.

Iron An essential mineral or trace element needed by the body to prevent anaemia.

Isoflavones Substances found in plant hormones that have a mild oestrogen, or anti-oestrogenic, effect in the human body.

Lactose Milk sugar, the naturally occurring carbohydrate found in milk.

LDL Low-density lipoprotein, a type of cholesterol that is harmful to the body.

Lecithin Fatty substance that emulsifies fats for transport in the blood.

Lignan A phytochemical with an antioxidant effect and a mild hormone effect (like Isoflavones, above).

Lignin A type of dietary fibre.

Limonoid Flavone in citrus fruit with an antioxidant effect.

Linoleic Acid An essential fatty acid of the omega-6 family.

Long Chain Fatty Acid Essential fatty acid such as linoleic acid.

Lutein Type of carotene.

Lycopene Red pigment found in tomatoes, which has an antioxidant effect.

Metabolic Rate Rate at which the body burns energy.

Metabolism The process of chemical reactions by which food and drink are turned into energy.

Methionine An essential amino acid (a building block of protein).

Micronutrient Vitamins and minerals (or trace elements).

Neurotransmitter Chemical that transmits messages between nerves.

NSP Non starch polysaccharides, a term for fibre that recognizes it as a form of carbohydrate because it is fermented by gut bacteria and does not pass through the digestive system unaltered as previously thought.

Niacin Vitamin B3, needed in metabolism.

Nutrients Essential substances from food such as vitamins and minerals.

Oestrogen Female hormone.

Omega-3 and Omega-6 Fatty acids essential for many body processes.

Pantothenic Acid A B vitamin.

Pectin A soluble fibre in fruit and the substance that sets jam.

Phenols Antioxidants in fruit and vegetables.

Phytates Substances in plants that bind iron, zinc and calcium to reduce their availability to the body.

Phytic Acid A potential cancer inhibitor that can also inhibit absorption of minerals from food.

Phytochemicals, Phytonutrients Substances in plants that are beneficial to health.

Phytoestrogen Plant hormones including isoflavones.

Probiotic Beneficial bacteria that lives in the gut.

Pyridoxine Vitamin B6.

Quercetin An antioxidant that is found in tea, apples and onions.

RDA Recommended daily amount of a nutrient suggested for good health. The term used on food supplements governed by EU law (or whichever country the supplement was produced in). The RDA does not necessarily equate to the RNI (see below).

Retinol Chemical name for vitamin A.

Riboflavin Vitamin B2.

RNI Recommended nutrient intake, amount of a nutrient recommended by the UK government as sufficient even for people with high needs.

Rutin A flavonoid.

Selenium A trace element with antioxidant properties, particularly anti-carcinogenic.

Serotonin Brain chemical that helps control appetite.

Sodium Chloride Known as salt, essential for health but problematic in excess.

Stanols See Sterols.

Sterols A naturally occurring substance in animal and plant foods that can lower blood cholesterol.

Superoxide Dismutase A powerful antioxidant enzyme that neutralizes potentially damaging free radicals.

Tannin Substance in tea and wine with an astringent quality.

Thiamin Vitamin B1.

Trace Element A mineral such as iron, zinc and selenium, essential for health.

Vitamin Organic substance essential for health.

Xanthophyll Yellow carotene with antioxidant properties.

Zeaxanthin Carotene with antioxidant properties.

Zinc Trace element essential for health, particularly the immune system

index

Acknowledgements

Many thanks to chief recipe tester Susanne Beard and her family of sturdy and indefatigable eaters, Andrew, Dan and Simon. Thanks also to Ian and Anna for clearing their plates and to all the other willing volunteers whose frank comments are always helpful.

Special Photography William Lingwood
Home Economist Sunil Vijayakar
Executive Editor Nicola Hill
Editor Abi Rowsell
Executive Art Editor Rozelle Bentheim
Designers Maggie Town and Beverly Price
Production Controller Jo Sim
Picture Researcher Jennifer Veall
Indexer Hilary Bird

Picture Credits

All pictures Octopus Publishing Group Limited/William Lingwood
except Octopus Publishing Group Limited/**Photodisc** 8 top left, 14